Mental Health Literacy of Adolescents in Urban Ethiopia and the Effectiveness of Mental Health Curriculum Intervention Using Social Media

ACKNOWLEDGMENT

First and foremost, I would like to thank the Almighty God for giving me the strength, patience, health, and blessing to accomplish this doctoral study.

I would like to use this opportunity to express my deepest and heartfelt gratitude to my supervisor, Associate Prof. (Dr.) Manas Ranjan Behera and my co-supervisor, Associate Prof.(Dr.) Pratap Kumar Jena, for their valuable advice and direction. Without their indispensable advice, discipline, and continuous guidance this work could not have been completed.

I owe a debt of sincerest gratitude to Prof.(Dr.) Sudhir Kumar Satpathy, Director, KIIT School of Public Health. I have gained enormous experiences from him, which I will need to contextualize in the academic realm and other facets of my career.

I also owe a debt of sincerest gratitude to Prof.(Dr.) Sasmita Samanta, Vice Chancellor , KIIT Deemed to be University for her help whenever I asked for my inquires sometimes beyond the school autonomy. I have learnt humanity and integrity from you VC Maam.

I would like to express my gratitude to the RSC members for their insightful and helpful scrutiny.

I would like to express my gratitude to the KIIT School of Public Health faculty members and supportive staff members for their invaluable support and assistance. I am very grateful to Mr. Shraban Kumar Behera, Senior Assistant, KIIT School of Public Health, for his charming hospitality and the services he provided me.

I would like to take this opportunity to thank KIIT University and environ community for their charming hospitality. You people are very welcoming and friendly!

I would like to take this opportunity to thank the Ethiopian Federal Ministry of Innovation and Technology, the Ministry of Education, and Dire Dawa University for sponsoring me to pursue my Ph.D.

I would like to express my sincere gratitude to the Dire Dawa Education bureau, the school administrators, principals, and teachers in Dire Dawa.

I would like to express my deep appreciation to the authority of Haramaya University's College of Health and Medical Sciences, particularly Negga Baraki, for making it possible to get ethical approval in Ethiopia.

I am also grateful to all my teachers, from first grade to postgraduate level, who guided me to reach where I am today.

My special acknowledgment goes to Dr. Legesse Tadesse, Dean of the College of Natural and Computational Sciences. I am grateful for his guidance and inspiration throughout my life.

I owe a heartfelt thanks to all my friends who have helped me in my education and life course. I thank my friends Molla Fentie, Melaku Masresha, and Melaku Adinew for their insightful advice, support, and comments. I am very grateful to my dear friend Abdulaziz Dessalew, from whom I gained a great deal of knowledge and experienced incredible work ethics, compassion, and integrity since we became acquainted.

Without the support and assistance of my wonderful, lovely wife, Fantaye Melaku, it is unlikely that I would be able to complete my doctoral study. I would express my hearty gratitude to you, Fantish, for the outstanding role. The moral boost from my daughters, Sosina Hailemariam and Helen Hailemariam has been invaluable in completing this Ph.D. study.

Without the support of my brother Tadesse Mamo, who has been there for me at every stage of my accomplishments, it is incredible that I would have been able to complete this course of academic study. Thank you very much, Tade.

I want to express my gratitude to my parents, sisters, brothers, and relatives, whose support and contributions have been vital.

LIST OF TABLES

~ xii ~

LIST OF FIGURE

LIST OF ABBREVIATIONS

APA	American Psychiatric Association
ASDs	Autism Spectrum Disorders
CAMH	Child and Adolescent Mental Health
CCA	Cross-Cultural Adaptation
CD	Conduct Disorder
CES-D	Center for Epidemiological Studies Depression Scale
CI	Confidence Interval
CIS-R	Clinical Interview Schedule Revised
CMD	Common Mental Disorders
CMS	Composite Measurement Scales
CSA	Central Statistical Agency
CSI-D	Mini-International Neuropsychiatric Interview
d	The margin of Sampling Error
DALYs	Disability-Adjusted Life Years
DID	Difference-in difference
DSM-5	Diagnostic Standard Manual – 5
deff	Design Effect
EDs	Eating Disorders
ES	Effect Size
FDREMH	Federal Democratic Republic of Ethiopia Ministry of Health
FIM	Feasibility of Intervention Measure
GAD-7	Generalized Anxiety Disorder Assessment
GBD	Global Burden of Diseases
GHQ	Global Health Questionnaire
HBM	Health Belief Model
HIV/AIDS	Human Immunodeficiency Virus/ Acquired Immunodeficiency Syndrome
HL	Health Literacy
HLS-EU	European Health Literacy Scale
HLS-Q12	Health Literacy Scale 12 in Number
HLS-Q47	Health Literacy Scale 47 in Number
ICD-11	International Classification of Disease -
IEC	Institutional Ethical Committee

IHRERC	Institutional Health Research Ethical Review Committee
IAM	Intervention appropriateness measure
K10	Kessler psychological distress scale 10 in number
KIIT	Kalinga Institute of Industrial Technology
KIMS	Kalinga Institute of Medical Sciences
LMICs	Lower and Middle-Income Countries
MHL	Mental Health Literacy
MHLQ	Mental Health Literacy Questionnaires
MINI	Mini-International Neuropsychiatric Interview
MoCA	Montreal Cognitive Assessment
ODD	Oppositional Defiant Disorder
PHQ	Patient Health Questionnaire
PTSD	Postpartum Psychosis and Posttraumatic Stress Disorder
RCT	Random Control Trials
RR	Relative Risk
SCMs	Social Cognition Models
SDQ	Strength and Difficulties Questionnaire
SF-36	Short Form 36 Health Survey Questionnaire
SPSS	Statistical Package for Social Science
SRQ-20	Self-Reporting Questionnaire
SSQ	Social Support Questionnaire
TRA	Theory of Reasoned Action
TPB	Theory of Planned Behaviour
UNESCO	United Nations Educational, Scientific and Cultural Organization
UNICEF	United Nations Children's Fund
WHO	World Health Organization
WHO-5	World Health Organization Well-being Index-5
WHOQOL	The World Health Organization Quality of Life Assessment

TABLE OF CONTENTS

~ ix ~

Mental health is among the primary public health priorities interlinking with physical health and well-being; as the saying goes, "there is no health without mental health." Nowadays, the burden of mental health problems and disproportional suffering among the adolescent population is increasing compared to other age groups for multiple reasons. Mental health literacy, defined as knowledge, beliefs, and awareness of mental health issues, is a notable modifiable factor linking to immediate and intermediate mental health outcomes. Understanding adolescents' mental health issues and these modifiable determinants are essential to maintaining a healthy mental state and improving well-being and quality of life. However, evidence about adolescents' mental health, mental health literacy, and the socio-demographic effects were inadequate in low-income countries, Ethiopia included.

Schooling systems as ideal places and mental health curriculum as organized content has gotten attention in promoting children and adolescents' mental health. However, resource limitations and structural inequalities necessitate an effective and sustained mode and medium of delivery. In this regard, digital devices, apps, and internet platforms have become imperative more than ever integrated with adolescents' daily life providing golden opportunities. According to qualitative evidence, online health interventions have reportedly overcome logistical and physical challenges. Social media, for example, provides these opportunities and has evolved into an appealing platform for exchanging health information.

However, affordability inequality creates the digital divide and digital differentiation related to devices and/or internet access, digital/internet literacy, and skills. Likewise, content selection and scanty evidence about the quantitative effectiveness of digital/internet-based delivery mechanisms and related outcome measures have challenged adolescent mental health promotion. Hence, there has been a need for quantitative evidence about effectiveness and measures of perceived implementation outcome and factors influencing mental health curriculum intervention using digital/internet focusing on mental health literacy. Direct beneficiaries' voices and stories must be heard and shared with full consent and active engagement while maintaining ethical and privacy concerns of intervention programs in public health for its scaling up and sustainability.

The thesis aimed mainly to investigate (1) mental health literacy level, (2) the perceived mental health status; (3) a mental health curriculum intervention effectiveness using social media (4) perceived implementation outcome measures to improve the mental health literacy level of adolescents in Dire Dawa, Ethiopia. Therefore, the thesis is composed of two interlinked components. The study's first phase consisted of a survey of mental health literacy and the prevalence of mental health issues (emotional problems, conduct problems, hyperactivity-inattention, peer problems, and pro-social behavior). Furthermore, the relationship between these mental health issues and the impact of socio-demographic factors were evaluated. The second phase of the thesis focused on determining whether a mental health curriculum intervention using social media significantly improves adolescents' mental health literacy or not. It also examined positive implementation outcome measures.

The study was designed from the viewpoint of the revised theory of the integrated health behavior change model and theory of change. The first part of the thesis consisted of a cross-sectional study among adolescents in grades 5 through 12 at public and private schools. Multistage random sampling was performed. The calculated sample size was 565. From approached 934 potential participants considering design effect and dropping out, 751 participants filled the questionnaire. About 731 participants' were taken for the actual statistical analysis after removing significant missing responses. Data was collected using the mental health literacy questionnaire (MHLQ), Strength and Difficulty Questionnaire (SDQ), and the WHO-5 well-being index after cross-cultural validation in the study settings. SPSS version 25 was used to carry out the statistical analysis involving normality tests, analysis of variance (ANOVA), Chi-square test, hierarchical multivariable linear regression, binary logistic regression analysis, and descriptive analysis. The prevalence of perceived mental conditions (caseness) was performed using the original 3-band categorization taking cut-off scores at 80th and 90th percentile. The correlation analysis calculated the relationship between the strength difficulties scale scores and mental health literacy scores. Estimates used a confidence interval of 95 % ($p \leq 0.05$).

The second part of the thesis was a quasi-experimental design (before-and-after design with the control) from the viewpoint of the theory of change. The before-and-after difference in mental health literacy was performed between the intervention (n_1=77) and control (n_2=76) groups. Effect size and difference-in-differences models

(95% CI) were conducted alongside other descriptive analyses. Perceived implementation outcome measures and influencing factors were assessed.

The mental health literacy score was normally distributed (Skewness=-1.321, Kurtosis=2.804) with a mean score of 135.98 and SD=15.50. Compared to male adolescents, female adolescents had slightly higher mental health literacy levels (p<0.01). Parental education, school grade, and ethnic/cultural affiliation explained about 10% of the variation in mental health literacy. The strength difficulty cut-off score for the present study was slightly lower for total strength difficulty and hyperactivity scores than the baseline despite relatively higher internalizing scores.

A significant proportion of adolescents (15.9-28.4%) experienced mental health difficulties, with a significant relationship with some socio-demographic characteristics (p≤0.05). Prevalence of perceived mental health issues was higher and reflected in the total difficulties (15.9-25.5%), internalizing problems (14.9-28.4%), emotional problems (10.4-23.9%), and peer relationship problems (17.8-25.8%). Prevalence of depression ranged from 18.0-25.5% across gender and age groups, which was higher in 14-16-year-old females compared to males and other age groups. When compared to the upper secondary grade level, the mental health problems prevalence was significantly higher for females in upper elementary (AOR: 2.60 (0.95-7.10, p≤0.05)) and lower secondary levels (AOR: 2.73 (1.19-6.29, p≤0.05)). It was significantly higher among male and female adolescents who had either themselves or their family members used psychoactive substances (p≤0.05). Perceived mental health issues were not affected by age, parental education, or employment (p>0.05). The research found a substantial negative correlation between mental health literacy level and strength difficulties scores (p≤0.05). In contrast, mental health literacy and subjective mental well-being were positively correlated (p≤0.05).

The effect size and the difference-in-differences estimates of intervention effectiveness to improve mental health literacy were positive. Despite the age and gender disparities, the effect size was significantly more prominent in the intervention receiving group than in the control group (p≤0.05). The effect size was estimated by Cohen's d and Hedges' g values, which ranged from medium to large (d/g=0.429-0.767, p≤0.05) size. Despite school grade, age, and gender differences, the difference-in-differences estimate showed a significant effect (DID = 0.348, CI: 0.154-0.542, p<0.001). The intervention implementation program was evaluated as appropriate, acceptable, feasible, and satisfactory. However, socio-demographic characteristics and other multiple perceived factors such as individual attributes, resources, and family-related factors were reported to influence the intervention effectiveness and implementation outcome measures.

The present study has achieved the proposed research questions, hypotheses, and objectives through the viewpoint of the revised theory of integrated health behaviour change model and theory of change. These findings were consistent with existing theories and results of previous studies. The thesis supports the claim that an evidence-based mental health curriculum intervention program using social media improves adolescent mental health literacy. It has implied the importance and effectiveness of mental health curriculum intervention using social media for positive adolescent mental health promotion. Socio-demographic characteristics, individual attributes, and family and resource-related factors were reported to affect the intervention effectiveness and implementation outcome measures.

Promoting mental health through mental health literacy necessitates culturally appropriate intervention programs. Promoting mental health literacy to enhance adolescents' positive mental health should prioritize vulnerable groups and individuals who start perceiving mental health difficulties. It is essential to understand the effects of these differences in countries such as Ethiopia, which are examples of multicultural and multiethnic diversity. Hence, further qualitative studies should involve unfolding how and why these happen and understanding the remaining determinants.

The study has some inherent limitations. One of the study's potential limitations was the difficulty of generalizing study results to all adolescents because of exclusion criteria for the survey and intervention study. Social media contamination was a limitation, even though the due emphasis was given throughout the study. Another potential limitation was the lack of previously available reliable empirical evidence involving interventions of this kind, restricted quantitative comparison efforts, and a highly restricted approach to the conventional interpretation of the effect size.

Keywords: *Adolescence, mental health, mental health promotion, Health literacy, , Difference-in-differences, Effect size, Ethiopia*

CHAPTER ONE

INTRODUCTION

CHAPTER ONE

1. INTRODUCTION

This thesis introduction chapter discussed the general background, rationale, problem statement, objectives, research questions, and hypotheses. It has further addressed the conceptual framework of the thesis, the definition of key terminologies, the structural organization of the thesis, and the chapter summary. These subtopics under this chapter include the following sub-headings.

- Background of the Thesis
- Motivation and Rationale of the Thesis
- Problem Statement
- Research Questions
- Objective
  - General Objective
  - The Specific Objectives
- Hypotheses
- Conceptual framework of the Thesis
- Operational definitions of Key Terminologies
- Overall Structural Organization of The Thesis

Chapter Summary

1.1. Background of the Thesis

Mental health is a primary concern of public health interlinking to physical health and well-being throughout life; as the saying goes, "there is no health without mental health"[1]. Mental health is intricately connected to influences other health outcomes[2]. Adolescent mental health has become part of the contemporary public health and healthcare issues[3–5]. Nowadays, the burden of mental health problems and disproportional adolescent population suffering is increasing compared to other age groups for multiple reasons[3–5]. In Ethiopia, mental illness represents 11% of the disease burden[6], and about 17-23% of young people suffer mental health problems[7,8]. Mental distress was reportedly 21.6 to 63.1% for college students[9].

Schooling systems as ideal places and mental health curriculum organized content contribute to the universal mental health coverage of the children, adolescents, and youth populations. As a result, measures of positive adolescent mental health promotion and prevention of mental illness become among the priorities of universal health coverage[2]. These health promotion measures must consider the target audience's motivation, ability, and capacity to access, rehearse, comprehend, and apply health-related evidence and facilities[5,10–16]. These attributes combine to form what has been defined as health literacy[17–19]. However, mental health issues received minimal emphasis than physical health in the general model of health literacy, motivating the development of the mental health literacy concept initiated as a separate school of thought[17–19].

Researchers have demonstrated that mental health literacy concepts and its building blocks can affect mental health outcomes [17,20–23]. Existing evidence suggests a lower knowledge and awareness is associated with more inadequate mental health services, despite the insufficient data for adolescents affecting the mental health promotion-prevention efforts[24]. It is critical to comprehend determinants and their interaction with socio-demographic characteristics in promoting adolescent mental health[25–27]. However, evidence from the population of low-income countries, such as Ethiopia, is limited. Adolescent mental health in Ethiopia has worsened due to health inequities that have resulted in a mental health promotion-prevention gap[7,8]. These health disparities and the promotion-prevention gap necessitate intentional and targeted intervention programs. Hence, evidence about mental health literacy and understanding existing perceived mental health issues should be readily accessible to develop effective intervention programs.

Adolescent mental health is an essential focus of epidemiological mental health research [3–5]. Nevertheless, there has been a shortage of epidemiological data on the perceived mental health problems prevalence and related determinants amongst school adolescents and the Ethiopian context[28]. The existing reports are qualitative, and comprehension of the quantitative correlation between mental health problems and mental health literacy is required.

Adolescent health disparities exacerbate the promotion-prevention gap in mental health[25]. Intervention approaches characterized as innovative, effective, acceptable, feasible, appropriate, and friendly are being advocated to bridge that gap[5,29,30]. These approaches assume interventions in school settings using technological platforms to address these gaps effectively. Still, the available evidence is limited in this regard. Investigating the effectiveness of such intervention approaches using technologies such as social media as a mode of communication for adolescent mental health promotion is therefore critical. Understanding implementation outcome measures and influencing factors of these outcomes is also paramount[31].

As a result, this thesis aimed to assess mental health literacy and investigate the mental health issues of adolescents in connection to socio-demographic determinants and the correlation between perceived mental health issues and mental health literacy in urban Ethiopia. The researchers wanted to see if a social media-based mental health curriculum intervention improves adolescent mental health literacy and is accompanied by positive implementation outcome measures. The socio-demographic variables and self-reported barriers affecting the effectiveness and other positive implementation outcomes were evaluated.

The thesis is divided into two parts. Part one of the thesis includes a cross-sectional investigation of adolescent mental health literacy and perceived mental health issues, the correlation between mental health literacy and these perceived mental health issues, and the effects of some socio-demographic characteristics. Part two of the thesis consists of a quasi-experimental study on social media-based mental health curriculum intervention effectiveness (ES and DID) and the implementation outcome measures (acceptability, appropriateness, feasibility, and satisfaction). Perceived factors that influence intervention effectiveness and outcome measures were included.

1.2. Motivation and Rationale of the Thesis

Adolescent mental health has piqued the interest of public health professionals due to the unique nature of adolescence and as a critical life stage for mental health promotion[4]. Adolescence is a critical developmental stage evolving and extending from childhood to adulthood, and the onset of puberty marks the beginning of an independent and responsible role in society[32]. It is distinguished by crucial physical, emotional, cognitive, developmental, and learning changes[4,5,33,34]. Adolescence is a critical period of life with changes in health and growth and development trajectories as a unique moment of transition. Significant physical, dietary, and social transformations occur throughout this developmental period, and these factors influence the quality of later life[4]. These circumstances influence cognitive and social abilities, health behaviours that affect adolescent health, and health issues later in life[35].

As the saying goes, "there is no health without mental health"[1]; mental health is considered to be integrally linked to physical health and well-being, with multifaceted burdens[2]. The science and advancement of mental illness research are advancing. When combined with other physical health issues, mental health morbidity contributes to adolescents' poor living conditions[36]. Tobacco, alcohol, other psychoactive substance use, behavioural problems, injuries, malnutrition, HIV, violence, and sexual and reproductive health are linked to adolescent mental health issues[37]. As a result, there is an increasing demand for adolescents' mental health and well-being outcome measures to inform the public and policymakers regarding individual or service level health promotion and therapeutic practices. In this regard, the strength difficulties questionnaire (SDQ) and the mental well-being index (WHO-5) have been essential to meet the criteria of definite measures. In this thesis work, a categorical approach to measuring mental health issues was favored and used over the dimensional approach, which considers the concepts of "normalcy" and "mentally sick" as two separate spheres.

As a result, researchers assess the preserved mental health issues using the common Diagnostic Standard Manual – 5 (DSM-5) and International Classification of Disease (ICD-11) analysis, effective in previous studies published[38,39]. This approach is marked by the clustering of disorders based on what is known as externalizing and internalizing problems. Instruments with high validity are routinely used to measure the internalizing (depressive, somatic, and anxiety symptoms) and the externalizing groups (substance use, disruptive, and conduct symptoms). Furthermore, the well-being state was examined using the WHO-5 index, with lower scores indicating depression. The externalizing and internalizing problems are expressed by emotional, hyperactivity-inactivity, behavioural, peer relationship, and social problems[38,39].

Mental illnesses are more prevalent in adolescents[36]. The prevalence of mental health problems has reportedly been disproportionally higher among adolescents. Approximately 10-20% of adolescents and children worldwide have mental health problems[40–42]. In Sub-Saharan Africa, it affects 19.8% [CI:18.8-20.7] of adolescents and children[43]. Despite the little evidence, a few surveys in Ethiopia found that mental health problems affected about 17-23% of adolescents with several burdens[7,8].

Adolescents' cognitive and behaviour skills are linked to drug-related, school, family, and social factors determining their mental health outcomes during adolescence and later life [44]. Academic performance, class attendance, retention relationships, and social interaction reportedly affect the overall health and mental well-being[45]. Extreme school rejection, underachievement, family disturbance, aggression, and self-harming behaviour all obliterate the consistent quality of life[46]. Most adult mental health disorders start during adolescence[47,48], implying that they impact future generations[29,49]. Among the first concerns of public health professionals and researchers would be the investigation of adolescent mental health issues and associated factors as the primary target for successful health promotion. Personal bad feelings and psychopathology expression into illness effects were the focus of previously used mental health promotion interventions. A new positive mental health paradigm has emerged to promote mental health, a viewpoint termed "good mental health"[50,51].

The key foci of adequate mental health promotion have recently been characterized as dimensions and components of good mental health[50,51]. As a result, the traditional elements of mental health promotion have given way to a paradigm shift. Individuals' negative feelings and psychopathology expression as illness effects[52] have evolved into a new realm of mental health promotion. Protective psychological, cognitive, behavioural, and social assets are investigated in this new dimension[51]. Thus, mental health promotion conceptions have morphed into a new concept of good mental health[50,51]. It is constructed into individual cognitive skills, mental health literacy, health-seeking intention, perception, emotions, behaviours, family, and social skills. Practical approaches to promote these critical dimensions of good mental health, especially mental health literacy, on the other hand, are still understudied[50].

Person mental illness are better understood when people have more knowledge and awareness about their health issues[17,53]. An individual's capacity, ability, and motivation to make sound health decisions combine to generate what is known as health literacy[5,10–16]. These behavioural skills influence the quality of proper and rational health decision-making[54]. Mental health literacy is linked to these behavioural and skill changes, or the level of information, attitude, and beliefs about mental health issues[17,21,23]. Understanding adolescent cognitive, emotional, and behavioural attitudes and skills are critical for promoting adolescent mental health and prompt intervention. Health literacy refers to these cognitive characteristics of a person in general[55].

Public health programs increasingly focus on health literacy as both a resource and a risk factor. On the other hand, multidimensional constructions and notions evolve quicker [55]. It is one of the intermediate health promotion targets and outcomes (knowledge, attitudes, motivation, behavioural, intentions, and skills) that affect intermediate modifiable health determinates (healthy behaviour, lifestyle, and effective health services, as well as striving for a healthy environment) [10].

These factors influence other health outcomes, such as reduced morbidity, disability, preventable death, and enhanced social outcomes (equality of life, functional independence, and equity) [10,56]. The principles and contents of health literacy apply to all aspects of health, including mental health. However, mental health is not expressly addressed in this definition of health literacy[22]. It does not always match the unique requirements of its diverse views and attributes[22]. Mental health issues are frequently overlooked and given less attention than physical health issues[53]. As a result, Anthony F. Jorm and his co-authors[17] established the term "mental health literacy," which has since become a school of thought [17,21,23].

Individuals and the general public frequently inquire about the steps for disease prevention, early intervention, and treatment[18]. Mental health issues are unreasonably overlooked or, if not neglected and receive far less attention[53], that is not enough for full-scale and positive mental health promotion[18]. According to epidemiological studies, knowledge of mental health issues and a positive attitude are strongly associated with actual mental health services use, later mental healthcare, and favourable results [13,57,58]. Individual teenagers' low cognitive and social abilities and poor health behaviour have played a role in these mental health outcomes[13,58].

According to the integrated health behaviour change theory, mental health literacy should be associated with proximal and distal outcomes. It is crucial for mental health and happiness. "Health behaviour change can be facilitated by promoting knowledge and attitudes that strengthen self-regulation skills, capacities, and social facilitation" according to the integrated theory of health behaviour change (ITHBC)"[59]. A similar scheme emerged when this paradigm was applied to mental health. Mental health literacy is about the information, attitudes, and awareness of mental health concerns that improve help-seeking, intention, self-efficacy, and health behaviour, influencing long-term health outcomes and quality of life. As a result, mental health literacy moved from the general scope of health literacy to the scope of mental health context, which Anthony F. Jorm and his colleagues initially envisioned and coined[17]. Mental health literacy is a changeable factor linked to improved mental health outcomes[17,20–23]. Mental health literacy refers to how well a person understands mental illness, their risk factors and causes, and the available resources to help them[17,20–23]. It includes one's potential to recognize specific disorders and aspects of mental distress and attitudes that promote recognition, knowledge, and appropriate help-seeking[17–19].

According to a contextualized integrated theory of mental health behaviour change model, mental health literacy has both proximal and distal mental health-related effects[13,57–59]. Anthony F. Jorm and colleagues a refined inclusive definition for mental health literacy is "*the ability of an individual (1) to know how to prevent mental disorders, (2) to recognize when having a mental disorder, (3) to know about help-seeking options and treatments available, (4) to know about self-help strategies and mental health first aid skills, and (5) to support others affected by mental health problems*"[17–19,22].

Most adolescents report delayed help-seeking to get prompt mental health services[60]. A lack of understanding about symptoms and nature of mental health disorders and alternate sources of support could affect teenagers' low help-seeking intention and behaviour [48]. With this data in mind, the mental health curriculum[61] has paid particular attention to those with a lesser degree of mental health literacy.

Adolescent mental health literacy fosters well-being and positive mental health outcomes[29,49]. Adolescence is crucial for physical, cognitive, emotional, and behavioural growth[4,62,63]. It has been a critical time for teaching vital mental health behaviours since these changes affect other health-related behaviours, skills, and abilities[54]. Many mental health problems start or worsen during adolescence and even last until adulthood. Hence, the period of adolescence is crucial for influencing mental health literacy and health behaviour change, ultimately for mental health outcomes.

Nevertheless, scientific research reveals that encouraging healthy mental health in teenagers, preventing mental disorders, seeking treatment, and seeking help for themselves and others has received insufficient attention[18]. There is scant evidence about teenagers' ability to recognize mental problems, their intention to seek treatment, and their behaviour in seeking help[53]. In high-income nations such as the United States, Australia, and Canada, a limited number of groups have launched state-wide teenage mental health literacy campaigns[64–70]. However, mental health, particularly teenage mental health, has not traditionally been considered a public health problem in developing nations such as Africa. In Ethiopian public health discourse, health literacy, in general, and mental health literacy, particularly, have received minimal emphasis until recently.

Health behaviour and results are influenced by socio-demographic variables [71–73]. Economic, environmental, and socio-demographic inter-individual inequalities are likely to impact mental health issues and knowledge and awareness of mental health issues[74]. For instance, mental health literacy disparities were reported across gender among young Australians, with female participants having a better ability to recognize the mental illness symptoms than their male counterparts[75]. Understanding the links between socio-demographic variables and mental health literacy is critical for determining how these disparities affect the efficacy of materials to promote mental health in teenagers.

Digital technology has advanced and has a promising role in enhancing public mental health literacy, which is essential for various reasons[76]. Utilizing the internet and digital technology[77], peer support using mobile phone[78], and different other website-oriented interventions[77] has provided several potential advantages and benefits for both the service provider and healthcare professionals[79]. Adolescents' daily lives are increasingly entwined with online platforms. It has much potential, and it's affordable. The timely intervention with magnificent anonymity and secrecy eliminates barriers linked with stigma and intervention distance to promote help-seeking intentions and behaviour related to mental health problems[80]. As a result, it opens up new avenues for delivering therapies in novel ways to expand their reach and effectiveness.

Intervention is a deliberate, targeted action to improve desired outcomes and effects[81]. The theory of change (ToC) serves as the foundation for the intervention study in this thesis, combined with the integrated theory of health behaviour change (ITHBC)[59]. It is helpful because it explains various circumstances and events using conceptual and empirical evidence to show how interventions are supposed to function through changes and mechanisms)[81].

Due to the intervention, knowledge, attitude, aspiration, skills, and health behaviours all change. After reaching and reacting to a targeted group within a period of applying goods and services designed to bring about these predicted modifications, these finally change health and well-being status[81]. The outcomes (or effects) are expressed as proximal and distal outcomes in these sequences of results. Implementation studies frequently employ the theory of change[81]. It considers acceptability, feasibility, appropriateness, satisfaction, effectiveness, and unanticipated outcomes. Additionally, the intervention process is linked to external stimuli. The theory of change makes various assumptions in each prediction node for change, including assumptions of causal connection, reach, capacity change, behaviour change, direct benefits, and well-being[81].

In the viewpoint of the theory of change, newly emerging technology increases and helps establish a health literate population, enhancing the capability of individuals to utilize trustworthy health information to make decisions right and improve their well-being [12]. Online and mobile technology have become deeply ingrained in the lives of adolescents, offering enormous possibilities for mental health literacy intervention [80], increased secrecy and anonymity, and a reduction in fear of stigmatization. Adolescents and young adults utilize social media more than any other age group[82], allowing them to generate and exchange health-related information through virtual networks. Fortunately, Ethiopia has the fastest internet adoption rate, and teenagers increasingly use social media in their daily lives[83].

Adolescents' digital literacy and use of social media have increased as students' progress in school. However, there is a lack of research on the effects of social media interventions on mental health literacy and behaviour change, particularly in low-income countries like Ethiopia. The schooling system and places are thought to be ideal for promoting the health of adolescents[84]. Nonetheless, studies and reports are scarce about the mental health literacy domains and the use of social media for the purpose of improving mental health in the school system of developing countries, including Africa. Most importantly, health promotion in schools using internet-based health promotion in Ethiopia is almost non-existent.

Technology-based interventions in school settings to improve adolescents' mental health literacy are projected to be practicable, cost-effective, and long-term. The primary rationale for the thesis was a lack of first-hand evidence about the level of adolescent mental health literacy and prevalence of perceived mental health issues in Ethiopia, specifically in Dire Dawa, as the chosen study area, and the need to establish and evaluate the social media-based intervention effectiveness targeting mental health literacy of urban adolescents.

1.3. Problem Statement

Given the higher prevalence of mental illnesses in low-income countries, documented evidence on adolescents' mental health in Ethiopia is limited. In the developed world, regional and cultural inequalities exist in the determinants of adolescent mental health and mental health outcomes[24]. However, empirical evidence on the mental health literacy of teenagers in Ethiopian schools is sparse. The prevalence and increasing burden of adolescent mental disorders with the deriving disparities are linked to resource limitations[85]. A shortage of qualified health workers, facilities, and resources is also associated with mental health problems/mental disorders and inequities[9]. These constraints of the skilled health workforce, lack of finances, and mental healthcare facilities, such as psychiatric hospitals and mental health professionals, are significant challenges in Ethiopia[9]. Hence, public awareness and health behaviour toward mental health problems and the determinate factor are critical in such circumstances. Thus, adolescent mental health literacy and help-seeking behaviour are increasingly important[86].

Ethiopian health policy emphasizes mental healthcare rather than good mental health promotion, where patients must visit hospitals and health facilities after mental health problems or illnesses arise. As a result, evidence-based intervention studies are required to support mechanisms that enhance the mental health literacy of adolescents and the intention and behaviour to seek help [80]. Such intervention must leverage digital and technological platforms in this digital age[5,87]. These tools help the public understand mental health risk factors and help individuals make better decisions[12]. Comprehensive research combining mental health literacy status with intervention effectiveness studies conducted online is required for mental health promotion.

Despite insufficient research on mental health literacy, poor mental health has been increasing, with a higher proportion of adolescents suffering from multiple types of mental illness[88]. Adolescents suffer disproportionately from mental health issues compared to other age groups. The proportion of children and adolescents worldwide suffering from mental health problems is reportedly ten to twenty percent[40–42]. A meta-analysis of 27 countries discovered that a significant proportion of children and adolescents(13.4% (11.31–15.9%)) had mental health problems[89]. The global pooled meta-analysis found a prevalence of child and adolescent anxiety (6.5%), depression (2.6%), ADHD (3.4%), and disruptive disorders (5.7%)[89]. Due to well-known health inequities, low-income children and adolescents risk suffering from mental health problems[90]. It is even higher among Sub-Saharan African adolescents[43]. According to reports, around (13.6-15.0%) of Sub-Saharan African adolescents who experienced psychopathological difficulties (18.8-20.7%) had mental disorders[91].

In Ethiopia, mental illness represents 11% of the disease burden[6], and about 17-23% of young people suffer mental health problems[7,8]. Mental distress was reportedly 21.6 to 63.1% for college students[9]. Few studies exist on school adolescents' mental health, and empirical evidence was rarely available in Dire Dawa, one of the Ethiopian provinces where this study was undertaken. Adolescent mental health promotion and intervention initiatives are limited due to a lack of evidence.

A lower level of mental health literacy has reportedly contributed to inequity in adolescents' mental health and affects their mental healthcare services[92]. It is associated with the stigma that discourages children and adolescents from seeking help [48,93]. Adolescents with poor mental health have inadequate awareness and intentions to seek help[21]. These adolescents are hesitant to seek mental health treatment [86]. These barriers impede appropriate care and contribute to harmful behaviours such as substance abuse, increasing risk factors for the poor quality of adult life, and premature death[94]. **For these discrepancies, several factors are reported.**

There existed geospatial and cultural differences in the mental health literacy level of adolescents and young adults[24]. However, mental health literacy in low-income countries is often misunderstood[95] and usually ignored[95–99]—almost non-existent for Ethiopian school adolescents. According to UNICEF, about 69% of Ethiopians aged 5-17 lack health-related knowledge[8]. Sixty-five percent of them lack health information and participation. This evidence varied according to state, rurality, and urbanity.

Mental health is frequently disregarded and under-researched in low-income countries such as Ethiopia[96]. The lack of studies on mental health literacy impedes effective mental health promotion and contextual intervention toward positive mental health. One of the deriving problem statements for this thesis was the lack of evidence about mental health issues and mental health literacy of adolescents in Ethiopian cultures and settings.

There is a scarcity of quantitative data on adolescent mental health literacy and perceived mental health outcomes. The impact of socio-demographic determinants on adolescent mental health literacy has been overlooked[96]. As a result, this study examined the mental health literacy level and perceived mental health issues among Ethiopian urban school adolescents. Effects of age, gender, school grade, ethnic and/or cultural affiliation, and mother and father education levels were all investigated.

Some qualitative descriptions revealed mental health literacy and well-being linkage, despite the lack of quantitative evidence of the correlation between mental health literacy, mental health issues, and mental well-being[98]. The deficit in available evidence necessitates an evidence-based assessment of the association of perceived mental health issues, mental health literacy, and mental well-being. The researchers proposed to examine whether exists a substantial correlation between mental health literacy, perceived mental health issues, and mental well-being.

Empirical evidence about adolescents' mental health outcomes and the associated factors are predicted as proximal and distal outcomes of mental health literacy for integrated health promotion. Understanding how factors interact with socio-demographic parameters in an adolescent population is critical for developing focused and flourishing mental health promotion. As a result, multifaceted programs promoting positive mental health must emphasize information, beliefs, and attitudes to mental disorders, risk factors, help-seeking intention, and healthy behaviours. So that individuals can develop anti-stigma attitudes toward persons with mental health difficulties.

Several studies found numerous intervention tactics at the population or individual level, mainly through training programs to enhance mental health literacy, including internet-based intervention[70,86,100–102]. In this time of information communication technology, digital activities and platforms are critical for adolescent health promotion[5,87]. New technology promotes health literacy by increasing access to information and helping understand mental health risk factors and sources of healthcare services[12]. The online intervention best overcomes physical and logistical limitations for health promotion[30,103]. Thus, social media helps share health information contributing to change in healthy behaviours[29].

Adopting innovative technologies to improve good mental health in schools is considered successful and sustainable[5,29,30]. Implementing such a practice requires a team, proper communication channels, and delivery mechanisms[49,50]. Through these strategies, the adolescent can increase their social connection and resilience. These communication routes get beyond physical and logistical barriers[104]. However, such mental health promotion evidence and experiences outside of formal schooling are inadequate[49]. The evidence is scarce about the effect of technology-assisted mental health platforms such as social media in the Ethiopian context. The use of social media to promote positive mental health was supposed to be practical, acceptable, feasible, and favoured focusing on contextualized domains of mental health literacy[58,105]. Despite that, digital inequality and other problems that impede these efforts in low-income countries have to get due emphasis.

In low-income countries, Ethiopia included [104,106], social media-assisted mental health promotion lacked quantitative evidence. There was little evidence about implementation outcome measures and determinants of effectiveness and these anticipated intervention outcomes. Implementation outcome measures are poorly understood in low-income nations like in Ethiopia[106]. These implementation outcome metrics and their influences must be documented to create comprehensive intervention programs. Hence, evidence from direct users is required to establish effective health promotion interventions for fair and robust universal health coverage[107].

Therefore, the study has two parts, and it was restricted to Dire Dawa in eastern Ethiopia. The first part of the thesis focused on mental health literacy (knowledge, attitude, belief, and recognition) and perceived mental health issues and well-being among 11-19 years old urban school adolescents with the effect of socio-demographic determinants. It further studied the correlation between mental health literacy, perceived mental health issues (total difficulties and subscales), and mental well-being. At the same time, the second part of the thesis focused on an urban school of adolescents aged 15-19 years assigned non-randomly to an intervention or control group. This thesis did not cover autonomous and implicit motivation or implicit attitude. The other excluded factors from the thesis were biological, economic, and environmental factors.

1.4. Research Questions

1. What is Ethiopian adolescents' mental health literacy level in Dire Dawa city?

2. What is Ethiopian adolescents' perceived mental health status in Dire Dawa city?

3. What is the magnitude of correlation between mental health literacy level, the strength difficulty scale, and mental well-being scores?

4. What is the extent of the effectiveness of a mental health curriculum intervention using social media to improve the mental health literacy of adolescents compared to a control group?

5. What is the extent of perceived implementation outcome measures for mental health curriculum intervention using social media to improve the adolescent mental health literacy of Ethiopian adolescents in Dire Dawa city?

6. What are the self-reported influencing factors affecting the effectiveness and intervention implementation outcome measures of mental health curriculum intervention using social media to improve the mental health literacy of adolescents?

1.5. Objective

1.5.1. General Objective

The study aims mainly to investigate (1) mental health literacy level, (2) the perceived mental health issues, and (3) the effectiveness of an intervention of mental health curriculum using social media to improve the mental health literacy level of adolescents in Dire Dawa, Ethiopia.

1.5.2. The Specific Objectives

1. To examine the level of mental health literacy among Ethiopian adolescents in Dire Dawa and estimate the effect of some socio-demographic factors.

2. To assess Ethiopian adolescents' perceived mental health issues in Dire Dawa and the effects of some socio-demographic factors.

3. To analyse the correlation between mental health literacy level, the strength difficulty scale, and mental well-being scores.

4. To investigate the effectiveness of a mental health curriculum intervention using social media to improve the mental health literacy of adolescents compared to a control group.

5. To examine the extents of intervention implementation outcome measures for mental health curriculum intervention using social media to improve the adolescent mental health literacy of adolescents

6. To identify the self-reported factors that influence the effectiveness and intervention implementation outcome measures of a mental health curriculum intervention using social media to improve the mental health literacy of adolescents

1.6. Hypotheses

1. Adolescent mental health literacy has a negative correlation with strength difficulty scores[perceived mental health problem] ($p \leq 0.05$, 95% CI)
2. Adolescent mental health literacy correlates positively with mental well-being scores ($p \leq 0.05$, 95% CI).
3. Mental health curriculum intervention through social media significantly improves adolescents' mental health literacy levels compared to a control group ($p \leq 0.05$).

1.7. Conceptual Framework of the Thesis

The thesis is conceptualized into two interlinked parts (**Figure 1.1**). The first part of the thesis is framed based on the integrated theory health behaviour change [59], focusing on mental health literacy (knowledge, beliefs, and attitudes about mental health issues and ability to recognize mental disorders), perceived mental health status, and mental well-being. Furthermore, the correlation between mental health literacy and perceived mental health status and the effect of socio-demographic characteristics were examined.

The second part of the thesis is based on the theory of change[81]. The pretest and post-test scores were taken for intervention and control groups to evaluate the effectiveness of a mental health curriculum intervention using social media to improve adolescent mental health literacy, estimated by effect size and difference-in-differences. The secondary analysis focused on the four measures of intervention implementation outcomes: the acceptability of the implementation, its appropriateness, feasibility, and the satisfaction of the intervention participants. Further, we assessed the perceived factors affecting the effectiveness and extent of outcome measures. Therefore, this conceptual framework shows the scope of the study–what the thesis was about and what it was not.

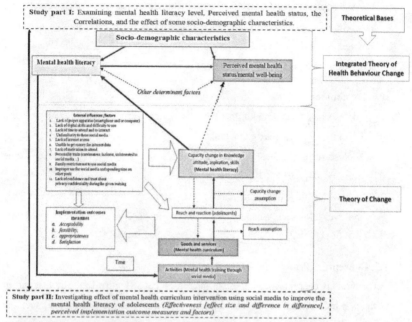

Figure 1. 2: Conceptual Framework of the Thesis

1.8. Operational Definitions of Key Terminologies

1. *Socio-demographic variables* in the present study context refer to a combination of social and demographic characteristics of the targeted adolescent population, including age, gender, religion, ethnicity, parental education and practices, ownership of smartphone, and social media use

2. *Adolescence* refers to a population group between 10 and 19 years of age divided into younger (10–14 years) and older (15–19 years)[108]. However, 11-19 were taken in this research, and adolescents exactly at the age of 10 were excluded from the cross-sectional part of the study, and the intervention study was conducted for older (15–19 years adolescents for sound reasoning and uncontrollable circumstances that are presented under chapter three in the section of inclusion and exclusion criteria.

3. *The mental health curriculum* is a guideline for promoting school adolescents' and young people's mental health that focuses on improving positive mental health outcomes.

4. *Mental health literacy* is individuals' knowledge, attitude, and beliefs about mental disorders, risk factors, and treatment options which aid their recognition, management, or prevention with its components, including (i) knowledge of about mental disorders and how to prevent, (ii) recognition of when a disorder is developing, (iii) knowledge of and attitude to help-seeking options and treatments available, (iv) knowledge of effective self-help strategies for milder problems(self-efficacy), and (v) first aid intention or skills to support others who are developing a mental disorder or are in a mental health crisis, and (vi) attitude to decrease stigma and enhancement of help-seeking efficacy to be assessed using the mental health literacy scale based measurement[18,19,109]. It is achievement tests and scales scoring on a continuum. Higher scores indicate better knowledge or understanding of a concept, and lower scores indicate limited knowledge, belief, and attitudes.

5. *Perceived mental health issues* refer to the perception of adolescents about their mental health condition. WHO defines mental health as "*a state of well-being in which the individual realizes his or her abilities, can cope with normal stress and can work productively and fruitfully*"[110]. Perceived mental health is a subjective measure of mental health.

6. *Strength and Difficulty Questionnaire (SDQ)* is a brief standardized, structured measure of mental health problems for screening for psychiatric disorders in children and adolescents. SDQ is a 25-item, 3-point Likert scale (0=not true, 1=somewhat true, and 2=certainly true) that measures emotional, conduct, hyperactivity-inattention, peer, and prosocial behaviour problems[111]. The total difficulties score computed as the sum of the first four subscales scores (the higher the total difficulties score, the more significant mental health problems)[111]. The fifth sub-scale reflects prosocial behaviour(the higher the score, the better the prosocial behaviour)[111]. The self-administered form of the Strengths and Difficulties Questionnaire was used for this study over the parent, and teacher forms[111–113].

   a. *The conduct scale* is a subscale of the total difficulties score obtained from the sum of five items (disobedient, destroys, tells lies, fights, steals).

   b. *The emotional scale* is a subscale of total difficulties score obtained from the sum of five self-reported items (SDQ3, 8, 13, 16&24).

c. *Hyperactivity-inattention scale* is a subscale of the total difficulties score obtained from the sum of five self-reported items (SDQ2, 10, 15, 21&25).

d. *The peer relationship scale* is a subscale of the total difficulties score obtained from the sum of five self-reported items (SDQ6, 11, 14, 19&23).

e. *The externalizing scale* is the sum of the hyperactivity-inattention scales and conduct scales reflecting substance use, disruptive, and conduct symptoms

f. *The internalizing scale* is the sum of the peer problems scales and emotional problems scales reflecting the depressive, somatic, and anxiety symptoms.

g. *The total difficulties scale* is the combination of externalizing score (hyperactivity-inattention scales and conduct scales) and the internalizing score (emotional and peer problems scales).

h. Prosocial behaviour is a subscale of total difficulties score obtained from the sum of five self-reported items (SDQ 1, 4, 9, 17&20).

7. *Well-being index (WHO-5)* is a Likert-type scale with five points ordinal scale *(5=All of the time, 4=Most of the time, 3=More than half the time, 2=Less than half the time, 1=Some of the time, 0=At no time)*[38,39]. The cut-off score for the WHO-5 well-being index (WHO-5) predicting depression is when the raw score is below 13 out of the total 25 scores, or one has answered 0 or 1 to any of the five items outlined by the International Classification of Diseases (ICD-10).

8. *Correlation* in this thesis context is the analytical approach to determine the magnitudes and direction of association or correlation between mental health literacy scores and scores of perceived mental health issues.

9. *The intervention (treatment) group* is a group of adolescents who received the mental health curriculum using social media.

10. *The control (comparison) group is* a counter-comparative group of adolescents that did not receive a mental health curriculum.

11. *Effectiveness of intervention is* the extent of the magnitude and change in mental health literacy of adolescents compared to a control group following the mental health curriculum intervention using social media expressed by *effect size(ES)* [114,115] and *Difference-in-difference (DID)* [116].

12. *Effect size* is the sizes of an effect measured by the magnitude of the difference in mean score between an intervention and a control group mean score values. It's an estimation of outcome measure in practical intervention and impact evaluation studies using Cohen's d and or Hedges' g. [114,115].

13. *Difference-in-difference (DID)* is a regression analysis result that explores a time dimension of the data to define the actual effect of the intervention and counterfactual effect[116]. In this thesis, it was used to estimate the intervention's effectiveness in improving mental health literacy.

14. *Intervention outcome measures* are indicators of intervention success to understand the implementation processes for more comparatively effective implementation strategies[31]. In this thesis context, the intervention outcome measures are appropriateness, acceptability, and feasibility of the intervention. Moreover, the satisfaction of adolescents with interventions was included.

    a. *Acceptability of the intervention*: is the perception of participants whether the intervention met their acceptance, the extent to which they liked it, whether they found it appealing, and whether they found it welcoming, and assessed by using an acceptability intervention measure questionnaire encompassing these four items[117].

    b. *Appropriateness of the intervention:* is the perception of participants indicated by their response to the perceived fit, relevance, or compatibility of the intervention program measured by using the appropriateness intervention measure questionnaire 4 items covering whether the intervention seemed to fit its purpose, was suitable, applicable, and a good match[117].

    c. *Feasibility of the intervention:* is described as the perception of participant adolescents about to what extent the intervention program was successfully carried out. It is measured using the feasibility of intervention measure questionnaire eliciting four items to what extent the intervention approach was implementable, possible, doable, and easy to use[117].

    d. *Satisfaction* was measured using seven items: the quality of the intervention, whether it was desired, whether it met the needs of the participants, whether they would recommend it to others, how much it helped them deal with their problems, and how much they would like to repeat the experience [118].

15. *Factors influencing the effectiveness of intervention and the implementation outcome measures:* are perceived factors influencing the effectiveness of the intervention and implementation outcome measures that are assessed using a 5-point Likert scale.

1.9. Overall Structural Organization of the Thesis

The thesis is composed of two interlinked parts. The first part consisted of a survey of adolescent mental health literacy, the prevalence of perceived mental health issues, the correlation of mental health literacy and status of perceived mental health issues, and the effect of socio-demographic characteristics. Part two of the thesis consists of a quasi-experimental study on social media-based mental health curriculum intervention effectiveness (effect size and difference-in-difference) and the implementation outcome measures (acceptability, appropriateness, feasibility, and satisfaction). It also included perceived factors influencing intervention effectiveness and outcome measures.

The thesis contains six chapters. This introduction **chapter (Chapter 1)** describes the background of the thesis, motivation/rationale, the problem statement, research questions, objectives, hypothesis, conceptual framework, operational definitions, and the chapter Summary. **Chapter 2** is the review of related literature part of the thesis on previously published works on the theoretical, conceptual, empirical, and methodological evidence related to the study variables and contexts. **Chapter 3** presents the study materials and methods. Study settings/area, study population, study design, sample size determination, sampling procedures, exclusion and inclusion criteria, data collection tools, data collection processes, intervention procedures, and statistical analysis are the subtopics described in detail in this chapter for both parts of the thesis. **Chapter 4** contains the study's findings we published in peer review and Scopus/PubMed indexed journals including the second objective findings already submitted for publication. These findings are presented in tables and figures, along with brief reports. The descriptive and inferential results are reported in chapter 4 in the same sequence of objectives and research questions appearing in the published articles. **Chapter 5** focuses on the thesis's discussion, strengths, and limitations. In this chapter, the discussion was made on finding with previously published related findings on the theoretical, conceptual, empirical, and methodological evidence related to the study variables and contexts. **Chapter 6** contains the conclusion, implications, and prospects of the thesis. Lists of appendices follow the references list.

Chapter Summary

Mental health is a primary concern of public health interlinking to individuals' physical health and well-being throughout life; as the saying goes, "there is no health without mental health." Nowadays, the burden of mental health problems and disproportional suffering of the adolescent is increasing compared to other age groups for multiple reasons. Mental health literacy, defined as knowledge, beliefs, and awareness of mental health issues, is a notable modifiable factor linking to immediate and intermediate mental health outcomes. Understanding adolescents' mental health issues and these modifiable determinants contribute to maintaining a healthy mental state that improves well-being and quality of life. However, evidence about adolescents' mental health issues, mental health literacy, and socio-demographic determinants was inadequate in low-income countries, Ethiopia included.

Schooling systems as ideal places and mental health curriculum organized content contribute to the universal mental health coverage of the children, adolescents, and youth populations. However, resource limitations and structural inequalities necessitate an effective and sustained mode and medium of delivery. In this regard, digital devices, apps, and internet platforms have become imperative more than ever integrated with adolescents' daily life providing golden opportunities. According to qualitative evidence, online health interventions have reportedly overcome logistical and physical challenges. Social media, among others, offers health information exchange opportunities.

However, affordability inequality creates the digital divide and digital differentiation by limiting device and/or internet access, digital/internet literacy, and skills. Likewise, content selection and scanty evidence about the quantitative effectiveness of digital/internet-based delivery mechanisms and related outcome measures have challenged efforts to promote positive adolescent mental health. Hence, there has been a pressing need for quantitative evidence about effectiveness and measures of perceived intervention implementation outcomes and related factors of mental health curriculum intervention using digital/internet focusing on mental health literacy. Direct beneficiaries' voices and stories must be heard and shared with full consent and active engagement while maintaining ethical and privacy concerns to scale up and sustain health intervention programs.

The saying goes, "there is no health without mental health,"; i.e., mental health is integrally intertwined with overall health issues and general well-being, with multifaceted burdens. Maintaining a healthy mental state during childhood and adolescence is crucial since it influences an individual's well-being and quality of life far into adulthood. As a result, adolescents are the primary research targets on mental health, emphasizing epidemiological studies of mental health issues and readily modifiable determinants. Hence, mental health literacy has become identified among the prior modifiable factors as both a resource and a risk factor determining mental health outcomes.

It is of the utmost importance to understand such factors with the effect of the socio-demographics and how they interact with the mental health condition of adolescent populations to build focused and targeted campaigns that enhance mental health conditions. There is limited evidence regarding mental health literacy and adolescent mental health conditions. The quantitative correlation of mental health conditions with mental health literacy and the effects of socio-demographic characteristics in low-income countries, Ethiopia included, have been overlooked. Qualitative evidence showed that people with a lower degree of mental health literacy exhibit more severe adolescent mental health disorders symptoms.

The schooling system and schools have been thought ideal for promoting adolescents' and children's health[84]. It is generally accepted that interventions in the mental health curriculum that use social media are effective and these interventions have been connected with suitable implementation outcome measures. Nonetheless, studies and reports are scarce about the domains of mental health literacy and school-based mental health promotion using social media in developing countries, including Africa. Most importantly, health promotion and disease prevention in school settings using internet-based platforms in Ethiopia are almost non-existent. Hence, the thesis has focused on these contextual backgrounds.

The thesis is composed of two interlinked components. The first phase consisted of a survey of mental health literacy, the prevalence of perceived mental health problems, and relationships between these mental health outcomes among adolescents attending school in an urban area of Ethiopia (Dire Dawa), and the influence of socio-demographic factors. Part two of the thesis consists of a quasi-experimental study on social media-based mental health curriculum intervention effectiveness (ES and DID) and the implementation outcome measures (acceptability, appropriateness, feasibility, and satisfaction). It included unanticipated perceived factors influencing intervention effectiveness and outcome measures.

The thesis has focused on two broadly stated problems elaborated into thesis problems, the problem context of what's known, why these problems matter, and how the problems were proven. The proportion of adolescents suffering from mental illness and poor mental health has increased. Adolescents suffer disproportionately from mental health issues compared to other age groups. Documented data on mental health literacy of adolescents and their mental health difficulties and related intervention initiatives for adolescent mental health promotion in Ethiopia is limited because of insufficient study evidence. Hence, evidence about perceived mental health conditions, adolescents' mental health literacy, and the effects of the socio-demographic characteristic were inadequate in developing countries, including Ethiopia. Direction, magnitude, and statistical significance of associations of these variables were rarely examined. Adolescent mental health promotion has been challenged with content selection and scanty evidence about the effectiveness of digital/internet-based delivery mechanisms and related outcome measures. There is a need for such evidence despite of scarcity of quantitative evidence about effectiveness and measures of perceived implementation outcome and the determinant factors for mental health curriculum intervention using digital/internet focusing on mental health literacy.

Therefore, the thesis aimed to investigate (1) the level of mental health literacy, (2) the perceived mental health issues, and (3) mental health curriculum intervention effectiveness with some outcome measures to improve the adolescents' mental health literacy using social media in Dire Dawa, Ethiopia.

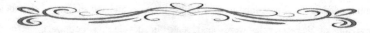

CHAPTER TWO

REVIEW OF RELATED LITERATURE

CHAPTER TWO
2. REVIEW OF RELATED LITERATURE

In this chapter, a review of related literature was conducted. This review of the related literature chapter comprises the previously published works on the theoretical, conceptual, empirical, and methodological evidence related to the study variables and contexts. The following sub-headings are covered in the review of the literature.

- Overview and search strategy
- Adolescence as a critical and essential time of transition in public health
- Understanding mental health as a subject of discipline
- Measurement of mental health
- Concept of mental illness prevention and promotion of mental health
- Adolescent mental health
  - Adolescent mental health problems
    - ✓ Prevalence of adolescent mental health problems
    - ✓ Adolescent mental health problems in Ethiopia
  - Measuring the mental health of adolescents
- Determinants of adolescent mental health
  - Effect of social and cognitive skills on the adolescents' mental health
- Health literacy and its notion for mental health context
  - Health literacy
- Mental health literacy
  - Concepts and constructs of mental health literacy
  - Measurements of mental health literacy
  - The integrated theory of health behavior change and mental health literacy
    - ✓ Proximal and distal outcomes of mental health literacy.
- Adolescent mental health and mental health literacy
- Evidence on adolescent mental health literacy level
  - Adolescent health literacy and mental health literacy in Ethiopia
- Evidence-based interventions and the theory of change
- Interventions to improve adolescent mental health literacy
  - Digital and online technologies for adolescents' mental health promotion
    - ✓ Social media platform for adolescent mental health promotion
  - Chapter summary

2.1. Overview and Search Strategy

This thesis aimed to evaluate and investigate (1) the level of mental health literacy, (2) the perceived mental health issues, and (3) a mental health curriculum intervention effectiveness with some outcome measures to improve the adolescents' mental health literacy using social media medium of delivery in an urban Ethiopia [Dire Dawa] aimed to improve the level of mental health literacy compared to a control cohort. The thesis has two sequential parts. The purpose of the first part of the thesis was to understand adolescents' adolescent knowledge, awareness, and beliefs about mental health issues termed mental health literacy. Simultaneously, it assessed the mental health issues from the categorical or clustering perspective of mental health (by setting a cut-off point). Mental health issues with the cut of points from strength difficulties score as normal vs. borderline vs. abnormal was categorized as internalizing problems (anxiety, depression, somatic symptoms) and externalizing problems (impulsive, disruptive behaviour, substance use).

Additionally, well-being status with WHO-5 index, lower scoring indicating depression (≤ 13) was considered. The former two clusters of disorders(internalizing problems and externalizing problems) are expressed in emotional, hyperactivity/inactivity, behavioural, peer relationship, and social behaviour problems[38,39]. The second part of the thesis aimed to examine and estimate the intervention effects of a mental health curriculum using social media as a delivery medium among school adolescents. The intervention implementation outcome measures and determinant factors were explored.

The scope of the thesis is delimited to some variables and population segments. Part one of the thesis focused on mental health literacy, the socio-demographic characteristics effects, and mental health issues and well-being. Other variables contextualized into the integrated theory of health behaviour change, namely autonomous and implicit motivation and implicit attitude were not in the scope of this study and the coverage of this review of related literature. This thesis does not address the socioeconomic, biological, social, and environmental-related determinants of mental health outcomes. Other anticipated proximal outcome variables, such as self-efficacy and help-seeking intention, were excluded. Precise behavioural control that includes decisions and actions was excluded. Part two of the thesis concentrated on mental health literacy change, intervention implementation outcomes, and the perceived contributing factors for the change and intervention implementation outcomes.

The review of related literature of this thesis was done by exploring up-to-date peer-reviewed articles. The most notable databases used include Cochrane library, PubMed, MEDLINE, EMBASE, ProQuest, ScienceDirect, Scopus, PsycINFO, Web of Science, WHO, and other national databases published from 2000 to the latest issue except for some theoretical and fundamental articles. The DSM-5 and ICD-11 manuals were referred to throughout the review of related literature.

The search for related literature was conducted throughout the study period. Searching the related literature was restricted to published literature in English. Keywords for the search were mainly focused on the following terms and their synonyms with the combination of different patterns. These most common keywords for the search were *"school adolescents," "adolescents," "mental health,"* "mental *well-being," "mental disorders," "mental illness," "health literacy," "mental health literacy," "mental health knowledge," "mental health awareness," "mental health attitude," "help-seeking," "self-efficacy," "mental health belief," "online intervention," "intervention outcomes," "online or internet," "social media," "intervention effectiveness," "Sub-Saharan countries," "middle and low-income countries," "Ethiopia," "health behaviour," "mental health promotion," "mental health services"* [22].

2.2. Adolescence as an Important Time of Transition in Public Health

Adolescence is a time of transition and a stage of life that spans the years between childhood and adulthood. It begins with puberty's onset and continues through the transition into an independent and responsible role in society[4,35,119]. It is characterized by critical physical, emotional, cognitive, developmental changes, and learning skills[5,33,34]. It is also a sensitive phase of life accompanied by the transformation of physical, nutritional, social, and environmental circumstances. Instead, these changes affect health and development and influence the quality of later lifetime[4]. These conditions determine adolescents' health behaviours, skills, and trajectories of health and development in later life[35].

These characteristics begin during the onset of physiologically normal puberty and the beginning of adulthood identity and behaviour. According to the WHO, adolescence is a developmental stage that occurs between the ages of 10 and 19

[120,121]. Nonetheless, the definition of adolescence is emerging and considers 10–25 years of age[4,35]. Epidemiological and socio-demographic transitions with the evidence of accelerated onset and delayed time of role transitions demand the need to redefine adolescence[4,35]. Despite evidence of these changes in patterns of change, the WHO definition of adolescence is maintained for this thesis.

Given these fundamental changes, adolescence harbors many risks and dangers[122]. Despite significant variations in the degree to which they are susceptible, every adolescent risks developing mental health difficulties[122]. Multiple findings showed that most mental health issues diagnosed in adults first appear during the adolescent years[47]. Many adolescents suffer from preventable chronic illness, infectious diseases, and disabilities from physical and mental conditions. About 97% of adolescent deaths occur in developing countries, two-thirds in sub-Saharan Africa and Southeast Asian countries[123]. Most adolescents(85%) with health problems live in these countries with noticeable health disparities[108]. At the same time, adolescence presents good opportunities for sustained health and well-being promotion establishing healthier adults and generations[35].

2.3. Understanding Mental Health as a Subject of Discipline

The topic of mental and psychological well-being and its nature is interdisciplinary, most notably dealing with psychiatric and psychological science disciplines with convergence sub-disciplines[124].The conceptual and methodological assumptions for mental health classification, measurement, and treatment in these two science disciplines have been parallel despite the need to integrate. To integrate psychiatry and psychotherapy in an effective and efficient way in clinical settings, a universally accepted definition of psychological disorders and an etiological model of mental illness are required.

Psychiatry prioritizes mental disorders' diagnosis, management, and prevention[125]. Pathoanatomical, neurological, symptomatic, and longitudinal courses emphasize mental illness. From a psychiatric perspective, medications or pharmacotherapy are prioritized over psychotherapy for mental and emotional disorders.

Diagnosis of mental health problems, treatment, and prevention are the prior considerations of psychiatry; pathoanatomical, neurological manifestations, symptoms, and longitudinal course of mental illness are the primary focus. From the psychiatric point of view, mental health issues or associated mental and emotional disorders prioritize the medications or pharmacotherapy followed by psychotherapy. Psychotherapy has been merging with pharmacotherapy. According to the psychiatrist, mental health involves understanding the interactions between the mind, brain, and body and how to use psychotherapy, medications, and the two together. At the same time, psychology focuses on emotional, relational, or behavioural challenges considering psychotherapy as a treatment. These therapies alter faulty behaviours, perceptions, emotions, and thoughts associated with specific disorders[124].

Mental health promotion from a public health point of view has emerged into domains of good mental health that encompass the epidemiologic and clinical practices collectively focusing on a population level[51]. It focused on mental health promotion and mental illness/disorders prevention. Positive mental health promotion strengthens the core domains of good mental health and its additional role in enhancing capacity and improving mental healthcare systems. The central core domains of good mental health include (1) mental health literacy, (2) attitude towards mental disorders, (3) self-perceptions and values, (4) cognitive skills, (5) academic/occupational performance, (6) emotions,(7) behaviours, (8) self-management strategies, (9) social skills, (10) family relationships, (11) physical health, (12) sexual health, and (13)quality of life that such a scope reflecting the motto that "there is no health without mental health"[51].

Studying mental health discipline and its conceptualization has numerous viewpoints. These main conceptualization perspectives include (1) dimensional, (2) categorical, (3) hierarchical,(4) neurobiological, (5) neuropsychological, (6) phenomenological, (7) idiographic, and (8) psychodynamic or psychological formulation perspectives. Existing arguments on explaining a mental illness as a cluster of symptoms or a single and defined phenomenon have brought the concept of categorical vs. dimensional approaches. Along with these approaches, causal explanation and psychiatric or psychological understanding of a particular disorder become one of the pinpoints for the selection of methodologies of mental health research. In this thesis work, a categorical approach(by setting a cut-off point) to measuring mental health issues was favored and used over the dimensional approach, which considers the concepts of "normalcy" and "mentally sick" as two separate spheres.

2.4. Measurement of Mental Health

Measurement and evaluation of mental health issues are more complex than measuring and assessing other health conditions[47,126]. Limited indicators and symptoms fail to capture the full spectrum of mental illness[47,126]. Lack of appropriate and flexible diagnostic guidelines and objective biological tests from which severity detection, mental health experience from intercultural differences, and complexity of social and psychological confounders make it more difficult [47,126].

The most commonly used measurements to investigate mental health issues are gathering data, biological tests, diagnostic interviews with gold standards, and screening assessment tools[126–128]. The data are linked to hospital records, prescription information, demographic details, health history, psychologist attendance referrals from big data, social diagnosis, and police records[126]. The second mental health measurement is biological tests utilized frequently in clinical and psychiatric research using EEG brain wave monitoring system and advancing appliances, and other proxy measures of stress like the level of salivary cortisol. The third assessment or measurement method uses a gold standard diagnostic interview to assess a person's mental health level through trained clinicians' careful and professional psychiatric interview. The fourth is screening assessment tools essential in time and resources, limited conditions, and large populations. These measurement methods were developed and validated to assess specific constituents of individuals' mental health, similar to diagnostic interviews through due care for accuracy of the data is mandatory[126].

The broader notion of mental health considers individuals' subjective 'well-being' that has emerged over recent years. Mental health issues are often measured in terms of illness with the usual measurement tools in four approaches using the indicators or contexts based on mental health level and purpose of measurement or evaluation[126–128].

The most common validated screening assessment tools to measure perceived mental health issues are notably using (i) non-specific general psychiatric symptoms assessments[SDQ-25, CIS-R, K10, SRQ-20, GHQ, SF-36 MINI & K6], (ii) for depression assessment [WHO-5, CES-D, PHQ, GDS,] and anxiety assessment[GAD-7], (iii) for cognitive function assessment [CSI-D and MoCA]. The fourth approach to assessing perceived mental health issues mainly focuses on factors related to mental health. These can be briefly measured using tools; (a) mental well-being by

WHO-5, (b) social support by SSQ, and (c) quality of life by WHOQOL[126,127]. To apply one or a combination of these tools, researchers select the methods which one fits best depending on respondents, interviewers, quality of estimate and data collection methods like paper and pencil or computer-assisted, interviewer and their style or self-completion[127,128].

2.5. Concept of Mental Illness Prevention and Promotion of Mental Health

Disease prevention and health promotion have overlapping boundaries[129]. However, Public health practices in healthcare focus on primary, secondary, or tertiary disease prevention, depending on disease severity and access to healthcare facilities through the healthcare system's hierarchy[130]. Hence, preventive strategies target risk factors and must be implemented to be effective before the disorder's onset. Once the illness develops, preventative measures can reduce its severity, course, duration, and disability[131].

Primary prevention has been identified as universal, selective, and indicated prevention focusing on the general population[130]. In contrast, particular prevention is directed toward specific individuals or subsets of those significantly at higher risk than others[130,131]. Secondary prevention includes all treatment-related interventions to reduce prevalence[130,131]. Tertiary prevention involves reducing disability, rehabilitating patients, and preventing relapses[130,131].

When discussing mental health, the term "promotion" most commonly refers to "positive mental health," not "mental illness"[131]. WHO defines health promotion as "enabling people to increase control over and improve their health" [132]. Instead of relieving symptoms and making up for deficiencies, mental health promotion emphasizes maintaining a positive mental state and developing better coping mechanisms in individuals. Mental health is an absence of mental illness or positive mental health outcomes[133]. Therefore, positive mental health is the desired end result of health promotion interventions.

Promoting mental health encompasses any activity that aims to improve mental health and well-being in individuals and populations. The emotional, cognitive, and related experiences of individuals, families, groups, or communities can all be strengthened through mental health promotion. Preventative measures and promotional strategies are intended to have a distinct meaning for a particular subset of the population the program serves. The two approaches sometimes have the same activities leading to different results. For instance, an intervention for promoting mental health to elevate people's sense of well-being contributes to lowering the prevalence of mental disorders[134].

Individuals' characteristics and actions contribute to their mental health status, behaviours, lifestyle choices, coping abilities, and the quality of their relationships with others[135]. Social status, income, employment status, housing, education status, working conditions, good physical health, and access to appropriate health services are other determinants of mental health[136]. Promoting the individuals, social and environmental conditions, and interventions to reduce or avoid these risk factors are all ways that one can work toward the goal of preventing mental disorders and promoting mental health[134,137,138].

Integrating promotion and prevention in mental health care has several benefits. Targeting a disease's risk factors and early symptoms is essential to preventing mental disorders. In addition, promoting activities that improve quality of life of people and societies is an integral component of prevention. Despite the widespread acceptance of health promotion and disease prevention within public health, there has been a consistent failure to include mental health aspects within these endeavors. Surprisingly, mental health is not given a higher priority, given the clear evidence that there are strong links between a person's psychological and physical health. To effectively implement programs, policymakers and practitioners need better understand the connections between mental well-being and physical health. The ability of individuals to deal with the social world determines the extent of active participation, toleration of diversity, and mutual responsibility. These abilities are associated with positive early bonding experiences, attachment, communication, relationships, and feelings of acceptance. Individuals' ability to manage their emotions, cope with life, and maintain emotional resilience is directly related to their physical health, self-worth, ability to learn, and ability to manage their feelings [134].

It is common to practice to use the terms "good mental health" and "mental health promotion" interchangeably[139]. The outcome of positive mental health is good mental health. Hence, promoting mental health across the lifespan aims to improve well-being, competence, and resilience[140]. Mental health promotion is intertwined with factors that help protect against mental illness[140]. Some people are at risk for a specific condition due to a trait, characteristic, or exposure that increases disease or injury risk[135]. Good mental health is not necessarily the absence of these risk factors but mental well-being with competence and resilience[51].

Promoting mental health emphasizes the fundamental components of good mental health[51]. Fusar-Poli, P., and colleagues conducted a review and enumerated that "*the core* domains *of good mental health comprise (1)mental health literacy, (2)self-perceptions, and values, (3)cognitive skills, (4) academic/occupational performance, (5)emotions, (6)health behaviours, (7)self-management strategies, (8) social skills, (9)family relationships, (10) physical health, (11)sexual health, (12)the meaning of life, and (13)quality of life*"[51].

2.6. Adolescent Mental Health

Health is "*a state of complete physical, mental and social well-being and not merely the absence of disease or infirmity*[32]. Well-being and mental health are integral parts of this definition. Mental health is inextricably intertwined with physical health and well-being[2]. A holistic statement affirmed that "there is no health without mental health"[1]. The science of mental disorders continues to evolve. Mental health morbidity contributes to impoverished living conditions of adolescents in combination with other physical health problems[36]. Alcohol, tobacco, and other psychoactive substances use, HIV, injuries, nutrition, sexual and reproductive health, and violence are strongly associated with adolescent mental health[37].

Promoting adolescent mental health is critical for various rationales[4,62,63]. To mention some of these rationales, the developmental nature of adolescence, public health scholars, and policymakers prioritize this age group. An increasing number of mental health problems and disorders manifest during adolescence[47,48,141]. There is a correlation between the prevalence of chronic illnesses and the mental health problems associated with them in adolescent populations[142]. The stages of physical, cognitive, emotional, and behavioural development that occur during adolescence are essential to an individual's long-term health and wellbeing [4,62,63]. These developmental processes shape behaviours and abilities related to one's health[54]. As a consequence, mental health during childhood and adolescence significantly influences the health outcomes of the subsequent generation [29,49]. In most cases, early intervention improves comprehension of health information [19] and ensures good health in the future[5].

2.6.1. Adolescent Mental Health Problems

Adolescents' health and mental health have become a significant public health issue in the recent efforts of healthcare, disease prevention, and health promotion [4,35,119,143]. Therefore, to achieve health, individuals must improve their mental health. The growing burden of mental disorders necessitates effective preventive and promotional measures[32].

2.6.1.1. Prevalence of Adolescent Mental Health Problems

Definition of child and adolescent mental health (CAMH) by WHO is expressed as the capacity to perform, attain, and maintain an optimal psychological and mental state of functioning and well-being in schools and within their community[144]. Mental disorder, alternatively called mental illness, has attributes of a change in how peoples think and feel, impeding their ability to perform daily activities[144]. According to the APA, mental disorders are clinically significant syndromes and disturbances of a person's cognition, regulation, emotion, and behaviour, reflecting a dysfunction and problem in underlying cognitive functioning manifested in biological psychological or developmental processes[145].

Noticeable disturbances of these attributes result in abnormal thoughts and problems with perceptions, emotions, behaviour, and relationships with others[143,145]: depression, bipolar disorder, and anxiety. Schizophrenia, substance abuse, psychoses, dementia, and other developmental disorders are among the most prevalent mental disorders[143,145]. Intellectual disabilities which have no distinct and complete boundaries from the other regarding symptoms, signs, and attributes are also mental disorders [143,145].

As explained in earlier sessions, adolescence is a state of the transitional stage of development described as multifaceted neurobiological, psychosocial, mental, and brain circuitry changes[146]. Hence, adolescent mental health problem is prevalent, affecting children and adolescents' optimal social relationships, psychological instability, and ability to care about themselves and others. It also impairs learning, positive interactions, and self-efficacy[41]. These problems are common in many adolescents with recognizable symptoms of physical, cognitive, or emotional expressions[40].

The WHO reported global mental disorders prevalence is 10-20% for children and adolescents [28]. Half of these disorders begin at 14 years of age[42]. Similarly, Most adult mental health issues start in adolescence[47]. All-world prevalence meta-analysis across 27 countries showed about 13.4%(CI:95% 11.3–15.9) of the global pooled mental disorders prevalence, indicating that the prevalence of mental disorders among children and adolescents is generally high[89]. From the study in general, depressive disorders (2.6%; CI: 95% 1.7–3.9), disruptive disorders (5.7%; CI: 95% 4.0–8.1), anxiety disorders (6.5%; 95% 4.7–9.1), and attention-deficit hyperactivity disorder (3.4%; CI: 95% 2.6–4.5) appear to be more prevalent worldwide, suggesting that other mental disorders should also be more prevalent worldwide[89]. According to a study based on self-reported SDQ scores, around 10.5% (5.8–15.0) of adolescents worldwide experienced mental health disorders, with more prevalent behavioural and emotional issues[147].

The adolescent mental disorders prevalence in Sub-Saharan Africa, where Ethiopia is included, was higher, which was reportedly about 14.3%(13.6-15.0%,95%CI) [91]. The majority of psychopathology was higher when using a screening questionnaire (19.8%; 18.8-20.7% 95 percent CI) than using instruments of clinical diagnosis (9.5%; 8.4-10.5% 95%CI)[91].

Table 2.1. **Prevalence of child and adolescent mental health problems in some countries**

Country/ location & [source]	Sampling method, instrument and (sample size) and	Target Age range	Mental health problems and (Prevalence)
Worldwide, Christian (Kieling et al.,2011) [28]	Lancet series, Global mental health 2	10-19 years	About 10-20% of children and adolescents worldwide suffer from mental health problems.
The global prevalence of mental disorders (Erskine H. E et al.,2016)[148]	Systematic reviews on Global The burden of Disease Study (GBD 2010) and (GBD 2013) from 187 countries	5–17 years	Mean global prevalence: 6.7% (Anxiety: 3.2%ADHD: 5.5%, CD: 5.0%, depression: 6.2%, ASDs: 16.1%, EDs: 4.4%).
Europe (Viviane K. et al, 2015) [149]	Systematic Randomization form parents and teachers of children(n=9084) from about 7 countries(Germany, Romania, Turkey, Bulgaria, Netherlands, Italy, and Lithuania)	6 to 11 years	School Children Mental Health in Europe. Average requiring some sort of mental health care (9.9%)' (Germany, Romania, Turkey, Bulgaria, Netherlands, Italy, and Lithuania)
USA(Wenhua Lu., 2017)[150]	Survey on children's health nationally (n = 85,637)	2–17years	The average lifetime and prevalence of mental disorders are 21% and 14.8%, respectively
China (Yang X., 2014)[151]	A two-phase cross-sectional study through parents and teachers, (n=8848)	6–17 years	Overall Psychiatric Disorders 9.49% (8.10–11.10%) and 15.2% two or more comorbid disorders AD: 6.06% (4.92–7.40), depression: 1.32% (0.91–1.92%), ODD: 1.21% (0.77–1.87) and ADHD: 0.84%, (0.52–1.36%).
India (Shilpa A.& Michael B. 2015)[152]	Review of ten years of evolution	10–19 years	The prevalence of mental disorders varied from 0.5% to 60%, with wide variation in the reported prevalence.
Australia(Julia D.et al, 2016) [153]	A web-based survey on Grades 7–10 from 21 secondary schools	12–16 years	Mental health problems of students scoring 'very high (19.0 %)
Russia (Helena R.et al., 2016) [154]	A two-stage design from rural and urban in the Tyva region of Russia (n=1048) from primary and secondary schools	9–15 years	Mental health problems affect 25% of adolescents, ranging from 40% of rural boys to 9% of urban girls.
Brazil (Carolina L. et al., 2018)[154]	Prospective cohort study (n = 4231) in early adolescence	11 years	The overall prevalence of psychiatric disorders (13.2%)
Sub-Saharan Africa including 3 studies from Ethiopia (Melissa A. et al,2012)[91]	Meta-analysis of 10 articles from 6 countries (pooled n=9,713)	0 to 16 years	Mental Health Problems 19.8 %(18.8% -20.7%)
Kenya (David M. N. et al,2016)[154]	Multistage cluster sampling, Youth Self Report (YSR) (n=2,267)	(10-13) years	The mental disorder of Children in primary school (37.7% (35.7–39.7 %).
South Africa(Jayati D. et al,2016)[155]	Cross-sectional associations (n= 1169)	14–15 years	School-attendees;Anxiety(16%), PTSD (21%), and Depression (41%). The relative risk (RR) of PTSD: 2.21. (95% CI: 1.73, 2.83). in black children, and CMD was 2.27 (95% CI: 1.24, 4.15)
Ethiopia National level (FDREMH,2013) [85]	Estimated to a national survey of Adolescents and youth	10-28 years	17-23%
Addis Ababa, (Desta M,2008)[150]	A multistage sampling of parents about their children (DICA-R) (n=864)	1-19 years	Epidemiology of child psychiatric disorders 17%
Dire Dawa(pilot study for this study (unpublished	Systematic Random sampling and using SRQ-20	(10-19 years	The mental disorder of School adolescents 37.8%
Ethiopian University students (Berihun A. et al.,2019)[9]	Meta-analysis of studies on Ethiopian Universities	18-25 years	Mental distress of students aged (21.6 to 63.1%)

A systematic review of studies in terms of global disease burden(GBD 2010) and (GBD 2013) from 187 countries revealed that mental health problems of children and adolescents 6.7%) and other mental disorders prevalence such as ASDs (16.1%), CD (5.0%), depression (6.2%), ADHD (5.5%, EDs (4.4%), and anxiety (3.2%)[148]. It is also expected to be relatively higher in other countries across the globe. For example, prevalence of national mental health problems of child and adolescent in Kenya[154], India[152], South Africa[155], USA[150], China[151], Brazil [154], Australia[153] and Russia[154] depicts comparatively its higher burden and frequency in Ethiopia[85,86,150].

2.6.1.2. Adolescent Mental Health Problems in Ethiopia

Ethiopia's youth's mental health has been recognized among prior national health issues. Despite the efforts to mental health promotion and prevention, prevalence remains incrementally[6,9]. In Ethiopia, mental illness and substance abuse burden keeps increasing as one of the leading non-communicable disorders, accounting for about 11% of the total disease burden[85].

Mental health problems of children and adolescents in Ethiopia are higher(17-23%)[85] than at the global level (10-20%)[28]. Substance abuse and mental illness have continued as significant public health problems, causing nearly an average of 1897 disability-adjusted life years (DALYs) per 100,000 people[156]. Substance abuse disorders (alcohol, khat, cannabis, linked mental illnesses, risky sexual behaviour) increase yearly [6,85].

Stigma, discrimination, human rights abuse and related mental health determinats and outcomes become common in our daily lives, mainly affecting children and adolescents[6]. In Ethiopia, the children and adolescents population's mental illness prevalence ranges from 17 to 23%, and university students' mental distress prevalence range from 21.6 to 63.1% [9].

2.6.2. Measuring the Mental Health of Adolescents

To measure mental well-being, the WHO Well-Being Index (WHO-5) is the most widely used instrument[157]. These five questions are sorted into six raw scores to choose from 0 to 5 points based on perceived mental well-being or quality of life presented about feeling towards the extent of one's spirits, relaxation, vigorously, freshness, and interest in things in daily life within the past consecutive two weeks. All response scores were added from the five different answers to obtain the raw score. The raw score ranges from 0 to 25; multiplying it by 4 gives a standardized score from 0 to 100[157].

A standardized score of 0 indicates the absolute worst possible quality of life, while a total score of a hundred indicates the best possible quality of life [157]. The most common mental health issues for this measurement are depression (ICD-10) Inventory. The cut-off score of the cases of depression from the well-being index (WHO-5) is defined as having a raw score of less than 13 or having to answer 0 or 1 to any of the five items. Therefore, a score lower than 13 indicate a poor state of well-being and warrants the possibility of depression (ICD-10). Several studies showed that WHO-5 has better performance screening depression than other questionnaires, regardless of combining aided clinical diagnosis[158]. It has demonstrated the best sensitivity and negative predictive value since it is perhaps the broadest of the measures.

2.7. Determinants of Adolescent Mental Health

Mental health issues and well-being depend on genetic, environmental, and behavioural factors[25]. For multiple reasons, adolescents are among the most important groups for mental health studies. Adolescence is key to physical, emotional, and cognitive progress. Fundamentally, mental, physical, and emotional developmental processes evolve during adolescence shaping health-related behaviors and skills **(Figure 2.1)**. Public health perspectives emphasize health information during early childhood, which would help in later life[4]. Another reason to focus on adolescent health promotion is the chronicity of mental health[4,5,33,34]. Some are fixed and permanent, while others can be changeable, promoting and maintaining better mental health (resilience factors) or worsening conditions (risk factors) [32]. Understanding these factors helps as a basis to design public mental health programs through effective interventions boosting protective factors and reducing the risk factors[25–27]. According to WHO, the most important determinants of adolescent mental health problems are substance use, forced migration, poverty, violence, harsh parenting, chronic illness, bullying, early pregnancy, sexual violence, early and forced marriages, and minority or discriminated group level [88].

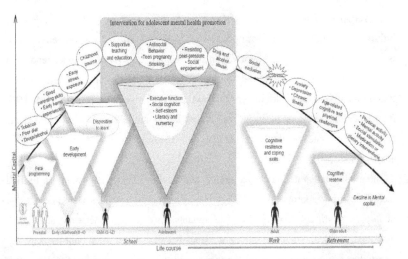

Figure 2. 1: Determinants of mental health outcomes in the life Course *(Adapted from Jenkins, R. et al. 2012*[159]*).*

2.7.1. Effect of Social and Cognitive Skills on the Mental Health of Adolescents

Social and cognitive skills (health literacy) and health behaviour as cognitive determinants of public health have become the central focus of epidemiological and intervention research in public health and behavioural sciences[16,160–162]. Social and cognitive factors mediate the relationship between socio-demographics, health-related behaviours, and health outcomes[11,54,163,164].

Social and cognitive factors are associated with various sets of cognitions related to health, referred to as health cognitions models determining health behaviour, termed a social cognition model (SCMs)[160]. Integrated social cognition models include (1) protection motivation theory (a revision and extension of the HBM; threat appraisal and coping appraisal), (2) the health belief model (perceptions of illness threat and evaluation of behaviours to counteract this threat), (3) theory of reasoned action/theory of planned behaviour(TRA/TPB(intention to engage in conduct and perceived behavioural control over that behaviour), and (4) social cognitive theory (goals, outcome expectancies, and self-evaluation)[160]. Social cognition models describe cognitive determinants and behaviour.

Cognitive determinants of health are primarily targeted health behaviour interventions. These interventions aim to improve mental and social skills, motivation, intentions, self-efficacy, and intention stability[46], which are interrelated and overlap with health literacy concept mediating variables [23], elucidating the influence of health beliefs and attitudes on health beliefs and attitudes on behaviour. It is the capacity, ability, and motivation to obtain/access, process, understand, and apply/use health information and services to make proper health decisions [10,11] framed with the three health dimensions and four cognitive domains[16,55,165–167]. It depends on the needs of an individual and the community, social capital and the health systems, and social factors that determine the health and health outcomes of the adolescent[11].

Integrating integrated social cognition and health literacy models into a unified theory targeting appropriate and effective interventions provides a comprehensive picture of modifiable interrelated determinants, mediators, moderators, and health outcomes [168]. In such conditions, a model is called the meditational model[162]. The independent variable causes the mediator[40], which also causes the dependent variable[56,169]. A mediation effect is an indirect/surrogate/intermediate/intervening effect. that also determines other health outcomes[170].

Mental health is a positive concept associated with individuals' and communities' emotional, psychological, mental, and social well-being. Hence, mental health is overlapped with overall well-being, and it is more than the absence of illness [171]. Good mental health signifies the joint statement *"no health without mental health"* [170,172]. In the lens of integrated social cognition models, adolescent age is an appropriate intervention period. Because adolescence is a time of sensitivity to early risk for the transition to dependence, including substance abuse[54]. The onset of disease and mental health dynamics determines the quality of adolescents' life. Thus, the adolescent age is an essential and ideal time for mental health literacy intervention to investigate the quality of life in the current and next-generation well-being[173,174].

It is imperative to focus on altering thoughts and beliefs most effectively and assess the causal impact of health behaviour change and cognitive skill, intention, and health behaviour change stability. A unified model/theory of health outcome determinants integrating health literacy and mental health literacy models with social cognitive models displays the inclusive public health spectrum and points of intervention (**Figure 2.2**)

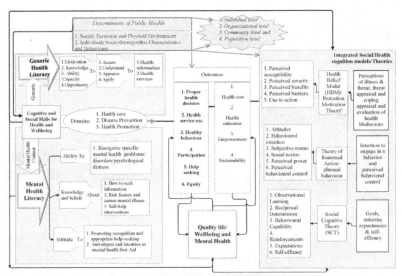

Figure 2.2: Interlinking health literacy, mental health literacy, and health outcomes with integrated social cognition models/theories (Adapted from *(Chinn & McCarthy, 2013; Hawkins et al., 2017; Number et al., 2012; Osborne et al., 2013; Sørensen et al., 2012* [16,55,165–167]).

2.8. Health Literacy and Its Notion for Mental health context

2.8.1. Health Literacy

Health literacy is an individual's capability/ability and motivation to access/obtain, process, understand, and apply/use information needed to make appropriate health decisions and healthcare services[5,10–16]. It is emerging faster as a multifaceted and developing construct and concept[55]. It is one of the intermediate health promotion targets and outcomes (knowledge motivation attitudes, self-efficacy behavioural intentions, personal skills) affecting intermediate modifiable health determinates(healthy behaviour, lifestyle and effective health services, and healthy environment)[10]. Instead, these factors determine other health outcomes, lower morbidity, disability, preventable mortality, and better social outcomes (equality of life, functional independence, and equity). [10,56].

It has clinical care and public health viewpoints[175]. Some authors have emphasized health literacy in the healthcare setting as a risk factor[142,176,177], and others consider health literacy an asset[16,175]. The health literacy conceptual model as a risk is frequently considered in clinical settings and practices, reflecting that low literacy impacts clinical care effectiveness. Concurrently, the health literacy conceptual model as an asset considers a broader range of backgrounds and perspectives and extends to more general applications outside health care settings[175].

Nowadays, health literacy most frequently emphasizes a public health perspective linked with knowledge and skills required in disease prevention and health promotion in daily life experience, including healthcare dimensions[16,178]. The European Union health literacy consortium has devised an integrated conceptual model for the current understanding of health literacy considered comprehensive and complete[16].

Surprisingly, some studies reported poor health literacy due to inequality in adult literacy [175]. A shift in demography and change in economic structure affects the health care quality and increases the epidemic of limited health literacy[175]. It seems to be contrary to modernization and advancement in the health care system; however, a reality that several studies are reporting as happening natural phenomenon. There must be complementary support-led strategies focusing on health education and empowerment in circumstances where social and economic inequities exist, resulting in health inequalities[179].

Efforts on inequalities as stated by 'WHO goal-'Health for All'[180] and UNESCO goal-'Education for All'[181] have complementary focus implicitly or explicitly towards improving health literacy. Hence, health promotion could be about ensuring that succeeding generations are better knowledgeable and skilled navigating health information and contributing to the healthcare system and services[182]. Health literacy is not only for an individual 'health benefit,' but it is also an asset for social benefits, community health empowerment, and social capital development [56].

Health literacy assessment and intervention programs during adolescence have been considered appropriate, compared to at the very early age or later in adulthood[5]. These interventions directly impact the health literacy level of later life as construction of setting in knowledge and behavioural patterns. These often occur significantly during adolescence through the transition into youth and adulthood[19]. Thus, focusing on reaching accurate and reliable health information for adolescents at this crucial time can help progress in lifelong healthier behaviour, enabling adolescents to exert their effort and take responsibility for every condition of their health and well-being[5,34].

Adolescents are frequently regarded as a healthy age group. However, more than 3000 adolescents die every day[93]. Others suffer from preventable chronic illness and infectious diseases and face difficulties of disability from physical and mental disorders[93,108]. Reports from lower and middle-income countries showed[123] that most adolescents live in these countries[108] and significant health disparities. For example, about 97% of adolescent death occur in these countries, of which around two-thirds (167 million) are from southeast Asia and sub-Saharan Africa[183].

Health literacy of the child and adolescent population is crucial and needs to be connected with the objectives and effectiveness of school health education. It is essential to see informed, capable, and motivated students who can make healthy choices and practice in all aspects of their daily life[5,34,184]. During childhood and adolescence, essential mental, cognitive, emotional, and physical change and development occur along with behaviours and skills related to health and well-being that increase sound decision-making[54].

Multiple reasons trigger pursuing health literacy research, practice, and exploring topics regarding adolescents' literacy, health, and well-being[5,54]. Globally, around 1.2 billion people(16.67%) are adolescents aged 10 to 19 years[42]. These adolescents face health challenges mostly from preventable or treatable causes. Severe and mild mental health problems, injuries, violence, premature and early pregnancy and childbirth, HIV/AIDS, drugs and alcohol abuse, micronutrient deficiencies, undernutrition and obesity, physical inactivity, tobacco use, and infectious diseases are among others[42].

Contextualization and operational definition of children and adolescents' health literacy in promoting health and well-being play a fundamental role in focusing efforts on the younger generation, a significant base for later life[142]. Combining mental health problems and chronic illness has become a growing and crucial public health issue among adolescents[5].

There is a literature gap in child and adolescent health literacy. The mechanisms through which literacy skills develop, improved assessment methods, the ease with which they can be accessed, and how factors such as schools influence literacy are all disregarded. Adolescents' interactions with health services and the drivers of their actions, behaviours, and decision-making abilities have received little attention[185].

With reasoning skills, mechanisms regarding adolescents experiencing and improving cognitive abilities that lead to an improved capacity to process information and think more advanced even about abstract ideas are identified as further research concerns[5]. First, public health efforts from such perspectives should prioritize early identification, intervention, and prevention[19]. Such priorities emphasize assumptions and practices of addressing health literacy at earlier ages and improve the interaction between adolescents and the healthcare system and their ability to understand health information, contributing to positive health outcomes even in their later lifespan[5].

2.9. Mental Health Literacy

2.9.1. Concepts and Constructs of Mental Health Literacy

The construct and content of general health literacy focus on all health domains; however, it does not always meet complex attributes of mental health[22]. Individuals and the public often try to prevent, intervene, and treat major physical diseases[18], unreasonably neglecting mental health issues if the case may be with much less attention[53]. Studies showed the need to promote mental health, prevent disorders, encourage treatment, and assist oneself or others with mental disorders[18].

Several studies have shown the limitations of individuals and the public's knowledge about recognizing mental disorders and how to prevent and when they develop [53]. The health literacy contextualized to mental health is called mental health literacy which was introduced and coined by Anthony F. Jorm in 1997 [17]. It is developed and conceptualized from the constructs and contents of health literacy (HL) models and literature [161] with modifications, defining it as *"knowledge and beliefs about mental disorders which aid their recognition, management or prevention"*[17–19]. According to Anthony F. Jorm and colleagues, mental health literacy incorporates recognition, knowledge, and attitudes about mental health[22]. It includes *"(a) the ability to recognize specific disorders or different types of psychological distress; (b) knowledge and beliefs about risk factors and causes; (c) knowledge and beliefs about self-help interventions and professional help available; (e) attitudes that facilitate recognition, and appropriate help-seeking; (f) knowledge of how to seek mental health information and g) avoidance of stigma and provision of mental health first aid"*[17–19].

2.9.2. Measurements of Mental Health Literacy

Measurement of mental health literacy is emerging and continuing in its development of contents, construct, psychometric properties, purpose, and contexts [186–193]. Measuring mental health literacy is mainly designed to determine individuals needing support and intervention and evaluate intervention effectiveness of implementation to improve mental health literacy[190]. It focuses on whether the public or individuals (i) recognize particular mental disorders, (ii) help-seeking intention for a mental disorder, (iii) attitude and belief towards the effectiveness of a particular self-help strategy, (iv) ability and attitude to mental health first aid providing helping hand for oneself and for whom with a mental disorder and (v) exhibiting and reporting and reducing stigma attitudes towards individuals who suffer from mental disorders[186].

The most common questionnaires featuring vignettes are used to describe attributes of symptoms and scenarios of a person[17–19]. However, it has multiple limitations for its time consumption during administration and psychometric property determination due to the lack of a scale-based scoring system and the difficulty of assessing all mental health literacy attributes addressing psychometric properties[190].

The commonly evolving and convenient mental health literacy measurement method is the scale-based measure, the Likert scale. It has been further adopted widely and developed through psychometrical, methodological, contextual, and cultural adaptations that are believed to investigate the mental health literacy attributes[190,194]. Other related and interconnected measurement tools within similar scope have evolved to evaluate knowledge and help-seeking attitudes, willingness and behaviours toward seeking help, mental health first aid, belief about intervention and prevention of mental health disorders, and anti-stigma attitudes[187,195–199].

2.9.3. Integrated Theory of Health Behavior Change and Mental Health Literacy

The integrated health behavior change theory provides concepts, definitions, and propositions interrelated to mental health literacy and its proximal and distal outcomes. The systematic view of these variables' relationship with causal pathways and determinant factors or situations by specifying relations among these variables explains and predicts proximal and distal outcomes (**Figure 2.5**). The model focuses on assessments and directs interventions that use best-practice improving positive mental health issues[59].

Constructs of mental health literacy and related outcomes could be adapted and conceptualized based on the integrated theory of health behaviour change (ITHBC). An integrated theory of health behaviour change is explained as "*fostering knowledge and beliefs, increasing self-regulation skills and abilities enhancing social facilitation, and engagement in self-management that change health behaviour. These changes can be the proximal outcome influencing the long-term distal outcome of improved health status*"[59]. For this thesis context, knowledge, beliefs, mental health attitudes, and ability to recognize mental disorders, termed mental health literacy result in behavioural change towards improving mental health and well-being[17–19]. Mental health literacy constructs are presented with hypothesized proximal and distal outcomes framed based on the integrated theory of health behaviour change (ITHBC) model (**Figure 2.3**).

The integrated theory of health behaviour change provides a set of interrelated concepts, definitions, and propositions in mental health literacy and its proximal and distal outcomes. It presents a systematic view of these variables' relationship with causal pathways alongside determinant factors specifying relations that can explain and predict proximal and distal outcomes (**Figure 2.3**). The model is essentially focused on assessing the status of these variables, then devising the use of best-practice interventions and implementing it to examine whether it improves mental health outcomes, especially adolescents' mental health [59].

2.9.3.1. Proximal and Distal Outcomes of Mental Health Literacy.

Mental health literacy outcomes can be seen as immediate, intermediate effects (or impacts) expressed as proximal and distal outcomes. The most notable proximal outcome results of mental health literacy are perceived behavioural control/self-efficacy and behavioural intentions. These proximal outcomes are health-seeking intention, actual behavioural control, action planning and decision, and health behaviours such as mental health-seeking behaviour.

Mental health literacy is essential to improve and often corresponds to help-seeking behaviours[187]. It reportedly influenced mental health services and perceived and expected treatment needs[88], indicating the need to integrate help-seeking mental health literacy. Anthony F. Jorm and his colleagues stated that changing knowledge is one thing and, in principle, not problematic. Being done time despites that changing heartily emotional reactions to practice caring and preventing mental disorders may be harder[23]. Parents, family members, peers, tutors, teachers, and schools significantly improve the mental health of children and adolescents.

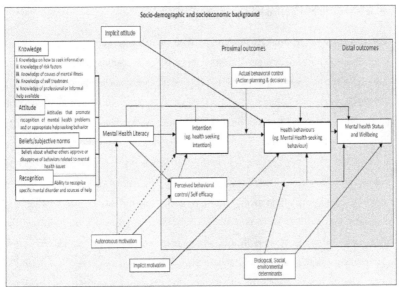

Figure 2.3: Proximal and distal outcomes of mental health literacy framed on integrated theory of health behavior change (ITHBC) model*(Adapted from Ryan, P., 2009*[59]*).*

Stigma, attitude deeply discrediting perception associated with public fear resulting from misunderstanding towards people having mental health problems as dangerous, consequently prejudice and discrimination in favor of others within social interaction and services[200,201]. Stigma linked to mental health conditions is much higher than stigma related to physical health problems[201]. These barriers hinder seeking help from informal and formal help sources reflecting the lower awareness and poor mental health literacy[90].

On the contrary, stigma has a tremendous effect on help-seeking behaviour. It isolates sufferers from their societal roles[202], a mostly known factor for late diagnosis and treatment delay for different mental health conditions[201]. Stereotypes, negative attitudes, and discrimination make the lives of people with mental illness more complicated and difficult, limiting help-seeking intentions and causing delay, treatment dropout, and poor medication adherence[202]. Several studies have revealed the link between poor knowledge and stigma[201,202]. Stigmatizing attitudes and low mental health literacy has been widely spread across cultures[202], implying that reducing stigmatizing attitudes should increase the mental health literacy of the public across various cultures and age groups, with special needs emphasis on adolescents[201].

2.9.4. Adolescent Mental Health and Mental Health Literacy

Several studies showed that the prevalence of poor mental health is increasing globally in the younger population[90] and the starting time for mental disorders is during adolescence or younger age[21]. These facts, but are not limited to, necessitate the need to focus on adolescents' mental health literacy. Adolescents worldwide suffer from poor mental health due to a lack of knowledge about mental health, a negative attitude, and poor help-seeking intentions[21]. When dealing with various mental health issues, they are often reluctant to seek help[86]. These adolescents who suffer from severe and debilitating mental health problems and difficulties lack seeking help intentions. Furthermore, these contribute to delaying appropriate help, aggravate the issues into different adverse health outcomes, and are accompanied by other exacerbating conditions like substance abuse, risky sexual behaviour prominent to further complications, poor adult life quality, and premature death[94]. The evidence and attributes of the problem in adolescents impose the need and interest in developing and executing investigation and evidence-based interventions that increase the mental health literacy of adolescents and behaviours related to help-seeking [86].

Mental health promotion stresses good mental health[50,51], including mental health literacy[51]. Initiatives promoting modifiable factors, such as mental health literacy, influence mental health outcomes in adolescents[17,20–23]. Hence, mental health literacy is, therefore, something that can be improved by using a mental health curriculum. A person's ability to recognize mental disorders and psychological distress, as well as their knowledge, beliefs, and attitudes regarding the risk factors, causes, and possible treatment sources for mental illness, are all components of mental health literacy (**Figure 2.4**). Appropriate acceptable, feasible, and effective mental health promotion approaches targeting adolescent mental health literacy in and out of school are limited, and their efficacy is inconclusive[49].

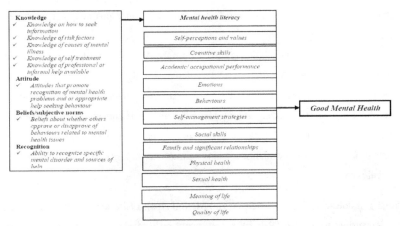

Figure 2.4: Core domains of mental health literacy and good mental health *(Adapted from Fusar-Poli et al., 2020*[51]*).*

2.9.5. Evidence on Adolescent Mental Health Literacy Level

Mental health disorders in adolescents remain increasing regardless of evidence-based interventions. Children and adolescents reportedly have lower mental health literacy levels reflecting the low treatment uptake rates. Mental illnesses are not properly understood or recognized by parents, who have limited options to seek help for their children and highly stigmatizing attitudes towards them[96]. Most youth needing mental healthcare are unaware and perceive it[84]. Deprived mental health literacy remains an obstacle and has become a challenging public health issue in developed and developing countries.

The importance of mental health literacy for childhood and adolescent disorders continues to be underestimated[95–99]. In the LMICs, mental health literacy is understood poorly or inaccurately, with scarce mental health services varying for different age groups, gender, and environmental settings [95]. Prevalence and level of mental health literacy vary across countries and population groups and various determinant factors despite limited studies on mental health literacy of adolescent populations, relatively fewer than on adults.

Research on mental health literacy in a university targeting students of western societies reported more significant gender differences-females had a higher mental health literacy level[203]. Less than 10% of participants believed they could list symptoms of a quarter of the less well-known disorders but could not translate to understanding them [203], implying that recognizing conditions does not guarantee adequate knowledge.

A population-based health literacy study from the Australian adolescent population using vignette showed that out of 1678 adolescents, only about 275(16.4%) had an adequate mental health literacy level, and 392(23.4%) intended to seek help[98]. Another study on stigmatizing attitudes from Spanish males revealed that adolescents who previously experienced mental health services/providers were higher [97]. Low mental health literacy prevalence remains an important adolescent mental health is a global issue.

2.9.5.1. Adolescent Health Literacy and Mental Health Literacy in Ethiopia

According to a 2016 UNICEF report, about 69% of children and adolescents in Ethiopia between 5-17 were deprived of health-related knowledge. Most of those living in households were deprived of health-related knowledge. The percentage of young adolescents deprived in the dimension was nearly two percentage points higher than children aged 5-14. However, the difference is statistically insignificant[8]. The proportion of adolescent girls deprived of health-related knowledge is significantly much higher(76%) compared to boys (64%)[8].

The proportion of children and Adolescents in Ethiopia deprived of health-related knowledge (69.3%) and deprived of health information and participation (65.7%) with slight variation across states and rural and urban settings (**Figure 2.5**). It was reported the highest in Somalia regional state for both deprived in health-related knowledge (92.5%) and deprived in health information and participation (84.6%) and lowest in the capital, Addis Ababa, 39.3% and 58.9%, respectively. The survey report showed urban residents had less percentage of deprived health-related knowledge (45.5%) and deprived of health information and participation (54.9%) compared to rural residents that were 72.7% and 67.2%, respectively[8].

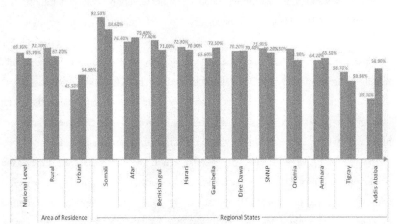

■ % Children and Adolescents Deprived in health-related knowledge in Ethiopia
■ % Children and Adolescents Deprived health-information and participation in Ethiopia

Table 2.5: The proportion of Children and Adolescents deprived of health-related knowledge and health information and participation in Ethiopia *(Extracted from CSA and UNICEF Ethiopia, 2018* [8].

2.10. Evidence-based Interventions and the Theory of Change

There is still a need for a methodological approach to generate evidence in various settings and for numerous kinds of interventions. The methods discussed earlier are all applicable, but each has advantages and disadvantages of its own. It is essential to differentiate between the following types of interventions by succeeding in a methodologically rigorous, multi-setting replication of the results based on methodological rigor. The evidence-based, effective interventions are ready for implementation; the probable effective interventions require more research; the unclearly effective interventions have not been adequately evaluated; the well-researched interventions are ineffective.

The following procedures have been arranged according to their intended population. A few examples are given to help illustrate these points. The direct effects of implementation and intervention studies affect the size and difference in the intervention and control group's mean score values. The absolute effect size can be calculated as the difference in the two groups' average or mean mental health literacy scores. Similarly, other intervention outcome measures/indicators are comparative effectiveness of implementation studies to change targeted behaviours and evaluate a specific intervention's efficiency or effectiveness in intervention studies[117]. These distinct implementation and intervention outcome indicators are appropriateness, feasibility, acceptability, adoption, fidelity, implementation cost, penetration, and sustainability[204]. These are necessary to determine whether or not the implementation was successful and monitor its progress and intervention efforts[117].

Most importantly, the intervention measures acceptability, appropriateness, and feasibility are commonly used in several studies [31,117,204–208]. Acceptability of the intervention is the implementation receiving members' perception that the given intervention practice provides satisfaction, assistance, or is agreeable. These are measured by using an acceptability intervention measure questionnaire[204].

In addition, the appropriateness of the intervention refers to how well it meets the perceived needs of a particular practice setting, provider, or consumer and how well it addresses a specific issue[117], measured by using an appropriate intervention measure questionnaire. The feasibility of the intervention is how well a new treatment, intervention, or innovation works in a given setting and is measured by using the feasibility of the intervention measure questionnaire[117,204]. These intervention measure questionnaires are in scale scores where although the cut-off score for interpretation is not yet available, higher scores indicate better outcomes. They are psychometrically and empirically tested for substantive or discriminate content validity[117].

Several studies on the acceptability, appropriateness, feasibility, and satisfaction of social media channeled intervention show various degrees and, in most cases, perceived the intervention positively[209]. For example, a similar study on smoking cessation intervention showed the highest participation, of which 81% commented on almost all the intervention content, positively[209].

2.11. Interventions to Improve Adolescent Mental Health Literacy

Mental health literacy has become a primary focus of intervention to improve the opportunities and ability for better long-term public mental health outcomes advancing early recognition, proper help-seeking and know-how for appropriate mental health first aid intention and skills for ongoing self-help and others facing stigma and difficulty of help seeking[21]. Several studies showed that mental health literacy could be improved using different intervention approaches at the population or individual level, mainly through various training programs [70,86,100–102]. Interventions that enhance early identification and help-seeking intention for effective treatment improve positive outcomes[84]. Mental health literacy research aiming to improve interventions to advance adolescents' knowledge, attitude, and ability is relatively limited despite the increasing number and types in various settings and diverse perspectives every year. These interventions aim to enhance adolescents' mental health literacy and focus on its constructs, resilience, and help-seeking skills, at least in four modalities. These modalities namely are (i) community campaigns whole at large, (ii) community campaigns focusing on children and adolescents, (iii) interventions schemes in schools, and (iv) training programs like adolescents' mental health first aid skills aiming at reducing stigma and help to seek about oneself and for others in such mental health conditions[21,210].

Adolescent mental health-promoting interventions can be realized in LMICs effectively in the community and school settings, resulting in positive mental health outcomes[190], and sometimes adverse effects may occur. A school is one of the ideal settings for promoting positive mental health and mental health literacy among young people[211]. A substantial number of study reports are available about school programs aiming at health promotion[23,192,212,213] designed to promote school adolescents' physical, behavioral, and mental health, among which mental health first aid is emerging in some countries[23,192,212,213]. School-based interventions positively affect adolescents' attitude, motivation, self-efficacy, confidence, self-esteem, coping skills, and behavioural well-being[99,214–216]. Comparatively, interventions for adolescent mental health in a community-based approach have also brought moderate to strong positive effects. They can be more effective in multi-component interventions for better mental and social well-being[211].

2.11.1. Digital and Online Technologies for Adolescents' Mental Health Promotion

Technology is a vibrant collection of practical applications and platforms for accessing health formation and is used for health-related educational interventions[5]. The emerging opportunity and potential of digital technology have given advancement and have a promising role in improving public mental health literacy with clear relevance for multiple reasons[76]. New communication technologies have become very important, helping individuals' access and obtain health information and assisting active involvement in health-related practices, decisions, and treatments. Hence, new and emerging technology advances the opportunities for the literate health public. It improves the public understanding of the risk factors and competence to acquire appropriate and timely health information and for proper decision making with analysis of 'true' knowledge about health and related issues[12]. Global and national efforts on literacy have been taken as one of the most fundamental actions utilizing technological platforms[87].

Utilizing mobile technologies such as text messages[74], mobile phone-based peer support, and the internet are becoming increasingly popular[77,78]. These various devices and web-based online interventions[77] offer plenty of potential advantages and benefits for both targeted recipients of the service and intervention and the service provider or healthcare professionals[79].

Traditional media such as community talks and discussions, pamphlets and print media, and the newly emerging platform technology such as mobile phones and the internet are used for interventions and improving mental health literacy[217]. Children and adolescents have also interacted with radio, television, social networks, and websites. These sources of information provide opportunities to access health information without specification to target population groups and health issues in specified conditions for measurable outcomes. Technologies such as online and mobile services have brought considerable potential and intervention opportunities to promote mental health literacy and good mental health in general. These technologies have evolved highly and interlinked with adolescents providing tremendous potential benefits. Because it is accessible, cost-effective, and timely with magnificent anonymity and confidentiality, reducing obstacles associated with stigma and distance of intervention improves help-seeking intentions and behaviour related to mental health problems[80].

The Internet remains an essential technology entity for seeking and sharing health and other information, accelerating its advancement and emerging platform exploring health information and daily communication in one's well-being[218]. The internet era has unquestionably contributed to disseminating and accessing health information for and through a significant portion of the global population[14]. The fundamental advantages and opportunities of the internet in day-to-day human lives are its easy access to information, avoidance of geographical restrictions, cost-effectiveness, and various supportive networks[219]. Emerging technologies on smartphones, social media, and other networking sites provide new opportunities for effective and suitable use in health promotion[220,221]. Health information, health behaviour interventions, awareness creation, and advocacy are essential. Public health efforts promoting youth resilience and coping skills reduce mental health risk factors and increase their well-being.

2.11.1.1. Social Media Platform for Adolescent Mental Health Promotion

Social media is the collection of various internet-based platforms and applications[197], such as Facebook, LinkedIn, Instagram, YouTube, Twitter, etc., used to exchange, share and collect information and create content [222,223]. The number of users is increasing rapidly. An estimated one-third (2.8 billion) of people use social media[224], of which more than one billion use Facebook daily [105]. It modifies the style of how people and organizations communicate[225].

Social media platforms have become helpful in exchanging health information [58,105]. It has played a tremendous role in improving health communication and education efforts[224] for health promotion, disease prevention, and management of diseases [222], promoting social connectedness in youth, and promoting resilience and well-being[105]. People interact on Social Media about health issues for health promotion, public relations, patient education, and crisis communication[226]. However, intervention studies on social media's public health issues are relatively new and under-researched [225].

Several studies showed the effectiveness of social media intervention trials on tobacco and alcohol cessation[227,228], adherence to medicine[229], self-management of chronic disease [224,230], and substance use[227]. More evidence included were mental health awareness and support[217,219,231], sexual health education and motivational messaging health [232], physical activity for health[233], nutrition [234,235], HIV prevention[229], sexually risky behaviour[232], weight loss[230], tobacco quitting[225], and hypertension awareness[236]. Common mental disorders (CMD) [1] and NCD[224,230] prevention practices use the internet and mobile-based interventions such as social media [224] as helpful and promising for cost-effective reaching a large population and addressing healthcare gaps[237] and overcoming potential challenges on-the-spot interventions[221,238].

Social media are ubiquitous in today's adolescents, representing social and digital media natives. They are fluent and tethered to digital devices, and social media[105], which create opportunities to enhance their relative independence, inspiration, abilities of decision making, emotional control, and peer relations, opening opportunities for exploration of their well-being and health are influenced by social determinants[239].

However, adolescents' limited preexisting health literacy may create conceptual misunderstanding of online information, increasing their risk of poor decision-making [237]. Cyber-bullying[105] and health information exchange determinants are other challenges[58]. Some degree of prior health literacy and understanding of the applicability of contexts is essential to learn effectively and to rule out incorrect information where better getting better and refined health information for better and proper health decisions[58,234]. Some researchers and scholars consider social media a double-edged sword [215], showing that adolescents' health literacy development must primarily emphasize health promotion attained by peers, teachers, parents, and adult support. Schools also need to educate students to use social media to improve health literacy which helps them develop positive health behaviours in their life course[237].

Interventions that use social media have concerns and multiple challenges. These challenges are connected to the small sample size, settings, measurement tools, participants' experience, and controls for comparison. validity for the statistical conclusion(extent of errors), internal(true effect difference), external(generalizability or adaptability), and construct validities(content)[225]. Social media interventions on public health issues are also a relatively new practice [225].

A mental health curriculum promotes positive mental health, improving adolescents' knowledge, beliefs, and attitudes regarding the recognition of mental disorders and the risk factors associated with them, as well as the awareness of available sources of assistance and information[20–22]. However, in the face of financial hardship, inefficiencies, and inequitable resource allocation, the mode of delivery has become a challenge. In low-income countries like Ethiopia and other African countries, inadequate health systems and structural inequalities necessitate novel approaches to mental health literacy improvement.

It is necessary to research populations of people with similar backgrounds and characteristics and to use the various communication modalities and strategies available for these specific target populations [49,50]. Schools are the best possible environments to improve the health of children and adolescents [84]. However, this approach's effectiveness, acceptability, appropriateness, and feasibility have been questioned[36], making it necessary to develop innovative collective strategies that use emerging communication technologies such as digital and online platforms. It is believed that these methods, which involve using schools as support platforms to establish direct communication channels with adolescents, are efficient, likely to last for a long time, and can be scaled up [5,29,30]. Text messages [77], mobile phone-based peer support[78], and web-based interventions[77] that take advantage of the internet and mobile technology offer many potential benefits for both the intended service users and the service provider. Multiple physical and logistical barriers necessitate using social media as a delivery channel[86].

Social media is widely used to exchange health information[58,105] and has become an integral part of adolescent daily life[240]. The highest percentage of social media users are those in their teens and early adulthood[82]. People can communicate with one another and share information and ideas via social media, including those that pertain to their health. Ethiopia currently has a rapid upsurge in internet expansion and an increasing number of social media user adolescents in their daily lives[83]. Internet use can increase social connectedness, resiliency, and well-being[67,105]. In developed countries, social media has successfully established itself as a communication medium for health promotion and intervention.

Chapter Summary

This review of related literature part of the thesis's primary purpose was to present and discuss the nature of adolescence, mental health issues, and concepts and measurements of adolescents' mental health literacy as the main focal point of the thesis. Hence, the topics of this review are organized, integrating, and bridging mental health issues and outcomes with the alternative of promoting adolescents' positive mental health, mainly on the mental health literacy determinants constructs and its proximal and distal outcomes.

In analogy to determining how wide to cast the net in catching fish, it was impossible to consider every available piece of research outputs; instead, more emphasis was given to central and pivotal peer-reviewed articles and published guidelines. The second part of the thesis focused on how interventions using digital and online platforms could be applied and how such interventions tend to be effective in diverse circumstances. The study was based on relevant theories contextualized into an integrated theory of health behaviour change (ITHBC) and theory of change (ToC). The series of topics addressed in this review of related literature align with the rationale of the thesis in terms of context, objectives, and the targeted study variables.

The integrated theory of health behaviour change is the topic and subtopics of the review of related literature. The nature of adolescence and adolescent mental health is a primary concern of public [mental] health. In this review of related literature, mental health literacy as a cognitive determinant was presented with its proximal and distal outcomes. Digital and online platforms, including social media for mental health promotion, were among the primary topics of this review of related literature. It also has entertained interconnected components of implementation outcome measures in the viewpoint of the theory of change contextualized into the context of the intervention part of the thesis.

CHAPTER THREE

MATERIALS AND METHODS

CHAPTER THREE

3. MATERIALS AND METHODS

This chapter provides the methodology for the thesis's cross-sectional and quasi-experimental studies. Hence, the thesis has consisted of two consecutive studies: cross-sectional and quasi-experimental (intervention study). The study design and analysis for both studies are dominantly quantitative. The chapter contains study settings/area, the population of the study, sampling, data collection tools, data collection procedures, and statistical analysis procedures. The following component subheadings are presented.

+ Study area and settings
+ Part I of the study (Cross-sectional study)
  ➤ Study design and methods
  ➤ Characteristics of the study population
  ➤ Sample size and sampling procedure
    o Sample size and sampling
    o Sampling procedure
    o Inclusion and exclusion criteria
  ➤ Study variables
  ➤ Data collection tools
    o Mental health literacy questionnaire
    o Strength and difficulty questionnaire (SDQ)
    o Mental well-being index (WHO-5)
  ➤ Adaptation and validation of the tools
  ➤ Statistical analyses
    o Analysis of mental health literacy level
    o Analysis of perceived mental health conditions
    o Correlations of mental health literacy score with strength difficulty scores and well-being index
  ➤ Ethical consideration
+ Part II of the study: quasi-experiment (intervention effectiveness)
  ➤ Study design
  ➤ Sample size
  ➤ Intervention materials
  ➤ Intervention procedures
  ➤ Variables and measurement tools
  ➤ Statistical analyses
    o Effectiveness of the intervention
      • Effect size analysis
      • Difference-in-differences analysis
    o Implementation outcome measures and the influencing factors
  Chapter summary

3.1. Study Area and Settings

This current doctoral study took place in the heart of Dire Dawa where the scholar has been working in Dire Dawa University. Dire Dawa city is known for its flagship characteristics of diversity in language, culture, traditions, and coexistence including foreigners determining health literacy, health behaviors and level of health outcomes reflecting the Ethiopian population across the country except for some peculiarities as Ethiopia is a country of cultural, geographical, traditional diversities. Therefore, Dire Dawa city was chosen for the present study.

Ethiopia is the cradle of the modern human being [241]. It has over 80 ethnic groups[242]. Ethiopia is the only African country that has never been colonized due to its resistance to European forces throughout the African conquest[243]. Ethiopia has the second largest population in Africa, the 12th most populous country globally, and the world's 27th-largest in size[244]. It has nearly 120 million inhabitants, making it the world's most populous landlocked country[244]. Ethiopia borders Kenya, Sudan, Eritrea, Somalia, Djibouti, and South Sudan. The capital city, Addis Ababa, is home to several global non-governmental organizations, including the African Union and different United Nations chambers and commissions for Africa.

Ethiopia is a country with a rising power status, but it is currently undergoing political turmoil and economic instability. It has one of the world's lowest GDPs per capita and significant structural difficulties. High poverty and a literacy rate of 49% make it a developing nation with a low per capita income and Human Development Index[245].

The recently reported average life expectancy for men is 56 years and 60 years for women[244], showing an increment over the past few years[245]. Ethiopia's population is 34.4% Oromo, 27.0% Amhara, 6.2% Somali, and 3.5% Tigrayan. Ethiopia has approximately 80 ethnic groupings (6.1%)[245]. Sidama (4% of the population), Welayta (2.3%), Gamo (1.5%), Afar (1.7%), Hadiya (1.7%), Gurage (2.5%), and others (12.6%) are other major ethnic groups[245]. Ethiopia is the only African country to employ the Ge'ez script[246]. Christians made up 62.8% of the population, followed by Muslims (33.9%), traditionalists (2.6%), and other religions (0.6%). Ethiopian Orthodox Christians make up the bulk of the country's Christians.

Ethiopia began establishing a policy in 2012, i.e., National Mental Health Strategy, which aims to improve mental health treatment[247]. As per the strategy document, mental health has to be included in primary healthcare[247]. However, the implementation of the strategy has only ended with little success [8]. Further studies conducted in Ethiopia revealed about 63.7% of general medical patients and 10.8% of community residents report anxiety and/or depression[248]. Stigmatizing attitudes, poor leadership and coordination, and a general lack of understanding regarding mental health impede effective mental health care.

This current doctoral study took place in the heart of Dire Dawa where the scholar has been working in Dire Dawa University. Dire Dawa is located at 9.5833 degrees (934'59.988" North) and 41.8667 degrees (4152'0.120" East) [249]. Dire Dawa provinces have been divided into two parts (a) city proper and (b) rural proper. The city proper is divided into nine sub-cities/kebeles, and the rural proper is divided into thirty-eight rural peasants' organizations (**Figure 3.1**). In 2018, Dire Dawa's population was 436,276, with 282,344 (65%) people living in the city proper[249]. According to recent data, 96,735 (10-19 year-olds) young population lives in the city[250]. Dire Dawa is notable for its language, culture, traditions, and coexistence with foreign dwellers. Ethiopia is a country of cultural, geographical, and traditional diversity.

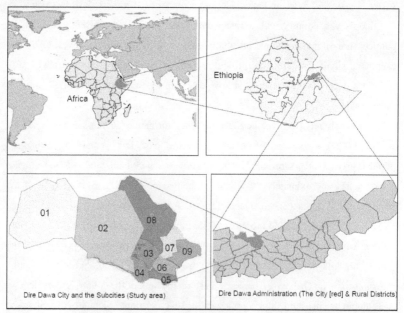

Figure 3. 1: Study area (Dire Dawa Ethiopia) (Numbers indicate the sub-cites)

3.2. Part I of the Study (Cross-sectional study)

3.2.1. Study Design and Methods

Part I of the study is a cross-sectional study design conducted in Dire Dawa, Ethiopia. About 934 participants were recruited, of which 731 respondents varied in gender, age, and socio-demographic characteristics completed the questionnaires.

3.2.2. Characteristics of the Study Population

The study participants were students aged 11 to 19 who attended urban schools. This part of the study focused on students from upper elementary (grades 5-8) and secondary (grades 9-12) levels in both public and private schools.

3.2.3. Sample Size and Sampling Procedure

3.2.3.1. Sample Size and Sampling

A calculated n=565 was the minimum sample size to estimate mental health literacy. An equation for cross-sectional study[251] was used assuming a 95% confidence level, a 5% significance level (α=0.05), a standard deviation of a normal distribution ($Z_{1-/2}$ = 1.96), the standard deviation of the measure in the population (σ=18.183), and a margin of sampling error (d=1.5). Hence, the following equation was used.

$$n \geq \frac{\left(Z_{-\frac{\alpha}{2}}\right)^2 \times \sigma^2}{d^2} = \frac{(1.96)^2 \times 18.183^2)}{1.5^2} = 564.514 \approx 565$$

However, about 934 samples were taken considering design effect (d=1.5), a 10% non-response, and dropout rate.

For the second objective as part of this study, which aimed to examine school adolescents' perceived mental health issues , the minimum sample size (n=560) was nearly equal to the above sample size taking the calculated margin of sampling error (d=0.04). The prevalence of self-reported mental health difficulty obtained from the pilot study of the same population was 37.8% (p=0.378)[252], taken calculating the sample size for the second aim of the thesis.

$$n \geq \frac{\left(Z_{-\frac{\alpha}{2}}\right)^2 \times p(1-p)}{d^2} = \frac{(1.96)^2 \times 0.378(1-0.378))}{0.04^2} = 559.673 \approx 560$$

After taking the same design effect (d=1.5) and a 10% non-response or dropout rate, a nearly equal maximum sample size estimation (n= 924) was obtained compared to the first objective sample size (n=934).

3.2.3.2. Sampling Procedure

The participants of the study were chosen using a combination of multistage sampling (schools, classrooms, and then individual students), systematic sampling (using a list of the students in fixed intervals of their roll numbers), and random sampling (using a list of the students in order of their roll numbers) methods (**Figure 3.2**). A total of 8 public and 7 private schools were sampled. Multistage sampling involves collecting data from schools, classrooms, and individual students. Schools, classrooms, and individual students all played a part in the selection process. The Dire Dawa Education Bureau was consulted to acquire the lists of schools and students. A random sample of public and private schools was chosen from each sub-city. Then participants of the study were selected randomly from each school, with the proportion of students selected based on the school's category and the grade level studied (**Figure 3.**2).

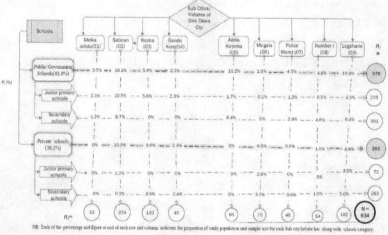

Figure 3.2: Proportion and size of samples from the eligible study population across sub-sites and public/private schools

3.2.3.3. Inclusion and Exclusion criteria

a. Inclusion Criteria

For the study's first phase, urban school adolescents aged 10-19 years old (grade 5 to 12) and actively enrolled in regular schools were considered. These students sampled from fifth to twelfth grade and attended junior and secondary private and public schools. A total of 7 private and 8 public schools were sampled.

b. Exclusion Criteria

The WHO definition of adolescence (10-19) was maintained despite excluding adolescents exactly at ten years of age for sound reasoning and uncontrollable circumstances. In Ethiopia, these adolescents below grade five are in the first cycle of elementary school, meaning they have not completed five years of education. Hence, adolescents at the age of ten were excluded despite the WHO definition (10-19). In Ethiopia, these adolescents below grade five have not completed five years of education; hence, they were excluded after the pilot study because they faced difficulty in recruitment due to the schools' nature and their challenges in understanding the consent and questionnaires. Another aspect of excluding these ten years old adolescents was the language barrier during data collection. The mother tongue languages of these adolescents were highly diverse, and they were unfamiliar with English. Adolescents from autism and slow learner schools were excluded. Further, night and distance program students were exempted.

3.2.4. Study Variables

The study variables for this part of the thesis are socio-demographic characteristics, mental health literacy, and perceived mental health (strength difficulties, mental well-being).

i. Socio-demographic variables include

- ➢ Gender
- ➢ Age
- ➢ School grade
- ➢ Ethnic/cultural affiliation
- ➢ Religious affiliation
- ➢ Paternal education
- ➢ Maternal education
- ➢ Paternal job
- ➢ Maternal job
- ➢ Self-experience with psychoactive substances use
- ➢ Any family experience with the use of psychoactive substances
- ➢ Parents practicing corporal punishment
- ➢ Adolescents report perceived worry about family problems

ii. The mental health literacy level comprised knowledge and awareness about mental health issues, symptoms, and risk factors, how to seek health-related information, how to avert mental disorders, self-treat, seek help options, and the availability of professional help. Health literacy includes belief/attitude to mental health problems, the symptoms and risk factors, the perceived ability to recognize specific disorders and when a condition is developing, and help-seeking efficacy. Attitude towards identifying mental health problems and attitude related to stigma towards mentally ill people and helping intention to others who may have symptoms of a mental illness or experiencing a mental health crisis are parts of the mental health literacy questionnaire.

iii. Perceived mental health issues are expressed as a self-rated strength difficulties score indicating the perceived mental, psychological, emotional, and behavioral problems and subjective mental well-being measured using the WHO-5 well-being index.

3.2.5. Data Collection Tools

The questionnaires were selected based on the COSMIN initiative guideline for measurement instruments[253,254] that explains procedures to assure questionnaires' validity and reliability. A comprehensive review of different peer-reviewed original and review articles and ready-made and published instruments were reviewed, along with concepts, contents, and scope of the proposed study objectives and conceptual framework[255–261]. Questionnaires were in composite measurement scales consisting of items/ scaled attribute questions. The questionnaires were developed in English and freely available[21,188,189,191,262–267]. However, psychometric properties for its reliability and validity for school adolescent populations were performed through pre-testing the questionnaires.

3.2.5.1. Mental Health Literacy Questionnaire

Utilizing the mental health literacy questionnaire(MHLQ), a measurement of mental health literacy was obtained, which preferred other frequently used tools validated for adults[268]. This MHLQ tool is freely available and validated for adolescent populations [21,188,189,191,262–267]. In the context of the current investigation, its reliability was evaluated using Cronbach's alpha and found to be 0.834. The version of the MHLQ contained 33 questions. Respondents were asked to respond to each question using a Likert scale that ranged from 1 (strongly disagree) to

5 (strongly agree), with strongly disagreeing indicated by 1, slightly disagreeing by 2, unsure about neither agreeing nor disagreeing indicated by 3, unsure about neither agreeing nor disagreeing is indicated by 4, and strongly agreeing by 5. The MHLQ contains awareness, knowledge, attitudes, and beliefs to assess adolescents' mental health issues[17,20–23]. The range of scores for the mental health literacy tool is 33 to 165. A higher score implies a better level of mental health literacy. Demographic information was collected along with mental health literacy.

3.2.5.2. Strength and Difficulty Questionnaire (SDQ)

The Strengths and Difficulties Questionnaire (SDQ) is a valid, rapid measure for emotional and behavioural problems worldwide[112,147,269–271]. SDQ is a 25-item, 3-point Likert scale (0=not true, 1=somewhat true, and 2=certainly true) that measures emotional(SDQ3,8,13,16&24), conduct(SDQ5,7,12,18&22), hyperactivity-inattention(SDQ2,10,15,21&25), peer problems (SDQ6,11,14,19&23), and prosocial behavior (SDQ 1,4,9,17&20) problems[111]. Adding up the first four subscales yields the total difficulties score (the higher the total difficulties score, the more significant the mental health difficulty)[111]. The fifth sub-scale of the SDQ reflects pro-social behaviour(the higher the score, the better the pro-social behaviour)[111]. This study utilized a self-administered questionnaire(SDQ-S[111,112]. The SDQ is widely used in resource-poor countries to measure mental health issues, behaviour, and emotional problems among children and youth in a collaborative setting. The SDQ-S is a validated measure, already translated into over 60 languages, including Amharic in the Ethiopian context., and used in over 40 countries to determine the mental health problems of children and adolescents[112,147,269–271]. The SDQ-S was found to be an effective tool for assessing children's mental health in a recent scoping review of 36 studies evaluating the SDQ-S in Africa[272].

3.2.5.3. Mental well-being index (WHO-5)

The mental well-being index (WHO-5) is an overarching expression for the quality of the various domains in the life of adolescents subjective to their mental and psychological well-being. It was evaluated using the WHO's well-being index, which consists of 5 items (WHO-5)[45,174,273–276]. It is a Likert-type scale with a five-point ordinal scale (*5=all of the time, 4=most of the time, 3=more than half the time, 2=less than half the time, 1= some of the time, 0=at no time*). The most common mental health issue is depression, often measured by the well-being index (WHO-5) outlined by the International Classification of Diseases (ICD-10). The cut-off score for the well-being index (WHO-5) scale was to predict depression. The raw scores below 13 out of 25 are taken as indicators of depression, or if one answers 0 or 1 to any of the five questions[45,174,273–276].

WHO-5 well-being index primarily assesses hedonic well-being, focusing on individuals' perceptions or feelings. It is about an individual's pleasant feelings frequently and having unpleasant feelings infrequently, as well as a general judgment that life is satisfying and makes up a person's happiness[277]. It is a perception of how well an individual life is going, getting things they want in life.

3.2.5. Adaptation and Validation of the Tools

Cross-cultural adaptation (CCA) was made on the selected questionnaire for the study context. The reliability and validity (content and face validity) tests were performed. The content validity and face validity were done by the judgment of a group of experts and input from the adolescents. An effort to improve the readability of the questionnaire was taken as a component of validity and reliability tests. The questionnaire's readability was addressed with wording and prepared in a hybrid of English with local languages following these subjective validity tests. Two independent translators did the translation into major local languages (Amharic, Afaan Oromo, and Somali) and were back-translated into English by others who had not seen the original one.

Based on the feedback of expert panels and the observation of pilot testing, the translation and validity test focused on the equivalence of the questionnaire mainly for its conceptual equivalence (cultural attributes with theory), item equivalence (relevance and acceptability), semantic equivalence (meaning attached to each item), operational equivalence (instructions, format of the scales, and mode of administration), and measurement equivalence (reliability and validity).

The reliability of the questionnaires was presented. Correlations assured reliability or internal consistency for the measure subscales and total scales. Accordingly, the test for reliability and validity was performed from the data obtained in this study. The reliability was acceptable that, The Cronbach's alphas were higher for the MHL questionnaire consisting of 33 items (α=0.838) and the help-seeking intention questionnaire composed of 12 items (α= 0.926). Cronbach's alphas for self-efficacy questionnaire consisted of 10 items (α=0.844), and the WHO-5 questionnaire with five items (α= 0.812) was higher and highly reliable. Face validity was performed by mixing things expressions with local languages with English. It was refined repeatedly until the administrators and participants agreed on the meaning to attain what it was intended to measure during pretesting. Content validity was assured by adapting previously validated measures for similar populations.

3.2.6. Statistical Analyses
3.2.7.1. Analysis of Mental Health Literacy Level

It is recalled that the objective of the analysis for mental health literacy scores was to examine mental health literacy and socio-demographics' effects on adolescent students. Version 25 of SPSS was used to conduct the statistical analyses. The formal normality tests (skewness and kurtosis) were preferred over the eyeball test to evaluate the normality of the data distribution. An asymmetric distribution is said to have skewness, while a peak distribution is said to have kurtosis. We use a skew index of absolute value less than two or a kurtosis index of absolute value less than seven to determine the substantial normality the present findings fulfilled[278].

The analysis of statistical significance was conducted at $p \leq 0.05$ and confidence intervals were calculated using 95%. Whenever there is a p-value less than 0.05, we consider the analysis outcome statistically significant using 95% confidence intervals. Socio-demographic characteristics were described concerning gender and mean age of study participants. Before computing the mean score for each individual, the MHLQ's negatively-keyed items (Q7, Q12, Q15, Q17, Q24, and Q26) were subjected to reverse scoring. Analyses of the socio-demographic characteristics and mental health literacy distribution were conducted with descriptive statistics. The mental health literacy score's mean, standard deviation, median, mode, range, interquartile range, skewness, and kurtosis were determined to understand the descriptive nature of the mental health literacy score of the sample participants.

Inferential analysis, viz. bivariate analysis, and multiple linear regressions were computed. Independent t-test analyses were performed ($p \leq 0.05$, 95% CI) among male and female adolescents to examine difference in mental health literacy. The variance in mental health literacy was tested using one-way ANOVA to evaluate the effect of socio-demographic characteristics. The relationship between socio-demographic factors and mental health literacy was examined using bivariate and hierarchical multivariate linear regression analyses were used to observe the separate and combined effect of these socio-demographic factors.

Estimates of regression coefficient and coefficient of determination (R^2) were determined with a significance of $p \leq 0.05$ and confidence intervals of 95% to evaluate socio-demographics' effects on mental health literacy levels. Before using the predictive regression model, there were two binary variables for each category; no equaled 0, and yes equaled 1. A comparison of mean scores for mental health literacy in male and female adolescents was performed using an independent-samples t-test.

3.2.7.2. Analysis of Perceived Mental Health Conditions

Like data analysis for mental health literacy, Stevens' measurement framework [265] was followed in handling SDQ measurement variables and scores. The data scores were treated as intervals. Aggregating individual item ratings computed Summated or aggregated mean scores. The cut-off score for mental health problems(cases) was defined in a collective setting adopting both original 3-band and new 4-band categorizations[279–281]. The cut-off score for the present study was described in a collective setting for the original three-band categorization.

A total score is determined by adding up the scores from each scale, ranging from 0 to 10. The summation of the emotional, conduct scales, hyperactivity-inattention scales scores and the peer problem scale which ranges from 0 to 40 is added to determine the total difficulties score. The cut of scores for the original 3 bands is defined by percentile into the highest first 10% (abnormal), the next 10% (borderline), and the remaining 80% (normal) as cut-off scores for total SDQ and the subscales[112,147,271]. The new 4 band categorizations into high, very high, slightly raised, and close to average in the same manner except high and very high scores fell in the first 10% (abnormal)[112,147,271].

The original 3 band approach was followed throughout the analysis. The cut-off for caseness was defined from the highest first 10%[112,147,271]. Descriptive statistics were employed to analyze the prevalence of adolescent perceived mental health issues (percentage). The Chi-square test was used to examine the statistical difference in prevalence across socio-demographic characteristics. An analysis of binary logistic regression was conducted to explore the effect of socio-demographic determinants (unadjusted and adjusted odds ratio).

3.2.7.3. Correlations of Mental Health Literacy Score with Strength Difficulty Scores and Well-being index

Bivariate correlations of mental health literacy were performed with strength difficulty scores and well-being index scores, respectively. The correlations of mental health literacy, WHO-5 well-being, and strength difficulty scores were examined. Correlation analysis was also done for the subscales of strength difficulties scores: emotional problems, conduct problems, peer problems, hyperactivity-inattention problems scores, mental health literacy, and mental well-being index.

3.2.8. Data quality Control and Bias Minimization

The effects of errors and bias were mitigated as much as possible. The questionnaires were prepared in hybrid English with participants' mother tongue, Amharic, Affaan Oromo, or Somali. Participants completed the questionnaire using the pen and pencil approach and were assisted and guided through the process. A comprehensive descriptive and inferential analysis was carried out objectively using standardized models broken down by age range.

3.3. Part II of the Study: Quasi-experiment (Intervention Study)

3.3.1. Study Design

Part two of the thesis was done by employing a quasi-experimental design that was a comparative investigation and analysis of the intervention (treatment) and the control groups before and after data collection (**Figure 3.3**). It was implausible that a randomized control trial could be carried out due to the high costs and numerous ethical considerations involved. Preventing contamination and bias during the intervention has emphasized assigning participants to intervention or control groups. In addition, it was challenging to control all known and unknown factors that could influence the intervention outcome. Hence, participants were recruited into geographically distant groups labeled as 'intervention' and 'control' groups based on the locations of their schools and areas of residency to minimize the extent of contamination and contact between the two groups during the intervention period.

3.3.2. Sample Size

Study objectives included comparing the change in mental health literacy scores from the pre-test to the post-test and comparing this between the intervention and control groups. Accordingly, the power analysis for this study was based on this primary aim. We determined the minimum sample size necessary for the study using systematic reviews of interventions for mental health literacy with its reported effect size of variance (δ =0.823). The standard deviation for two was 1.55[50]. The calculation was based on the assumption of confidence of 95% ($Z\alpha/2$ =1.96), power of 90% (Z_β=1.282), and type 1 error α=5%. A minimum of 146 participants (73 for each arm) were calculated using a frequently used sample size calculation for quasi-experimental studies[251].

$$n = \frac{2\sigma^2 (Z\alpha + Z1\_\beta)^2}{\delta^2} = \frac{2 * 1.53^2 (1.96 + 1.282)^2}{0.0.823^2} = 72.6506 \sim 73$$

Nevertheless, 213 participants from the study's first part (cross-sectional) met the inclusion criteria for part two (quasi-experimental) and were approached and almost equally allocated into intervention and control groups. However, only 156 from both groups those 77 participants for intervention and 76 participants for control completed the intervention and filled the post-test questionnaire (**Figure 3.3**). The pretest record of these participants (pretest score) was taken from their mental health literacy score obtained during the study's first part (cross-sectional).

3.3.3.   Inclusion and Exclusion Criteria
a.   Inclusion Criteria

For this quasi-experimental study, only 15-19 years of adolescents were included, mainly for three reasons. (1) Participants in the intervention study were required necessarily access the internet for social media use during the study period. (2) The maturity level of adolescents who can understand the intervention with the adolescents of 15-19 years age group. (3) Another factor was appropriateness to have the same intervention strategy across the narrow variation in age groups where the intervention was restricted on 15-19 age groups where maturity level of other 11-14 years adolescents is not up to the mark with the adolescents of 15-19 years age group.

b.   Exclusion Criteria

Adolescents 11-14 years of age were excluded for the following reasons. (1) In the Ethiopian context, adolescents do not have internet or digital devices. (2) The maturity level of these adolescents is not up to the mark with the adolescents of 15-19 years age group. (3) Another challenge was ethical and practical issues that adolescents aged 11 -14 years were unsure to understand the contents of informed consent to participate in the intervention study.

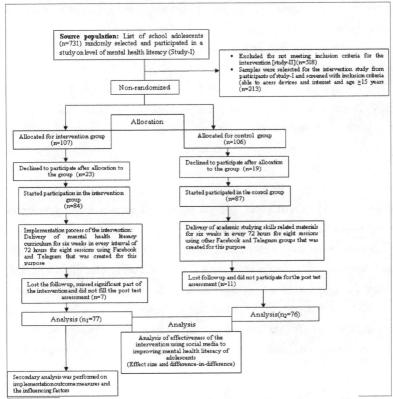

Figure 3.3: Flow chart of the study design for the quasi-experiment study.

3.3.4. Intervention Materials

The intervention material (manual) consisted of a mental health curriculum tailored specifically for adolescents. It was adapted from the school mental health curriculum guides already prepared for adolescents in Africa, Australia, and Canada to improve mental health literacy and first aid skills[64–70]. This was done to improve mental health literacy and mental health first aid skills. In order to accomplish the preparation and presentation of the intervention material for this study, a summary of the texts, figures, and case vignettes found within the manual was done.

The content of the intervention manual consisted of information on mental disorders and mental health problems and how to seek information. The manual included information on risk factors and protective factors, causes of mental illness, self-help and help for others, and information about professional or informal resources. Furthermore, attitudes related to promoting recognition of mental health problems and appropriate help-seeking behaviour, as well as recognizing mental health conditions, is among the primary constructs of the mental health curriculum.

3.3.4. Intervention Procedures

According to the inclusion criteria for the quasi-experimental part, 213 participants were identified from the first part (cross-sectional study). Pretest scores obtained during the cross-sectional study were used to compare the post-test scores obtained after the intervention. A pilot intervention was followed[282] to assess the intervention feasibility. Then a pilot intervention was followed to evaluate the intervention feasibility. However, only 156 from both groups those 77 participants for intervention and 76 participants for control completed the intervention program and filled the post-test questionnaire (**Figure 3.3**).

Reports showed that Facebook and Telegram were the social media platforms used most frequently by Ethiopian adolescents in the Dire Dawa region of Ethiopia[282]. Based on the pilot intervention outcome[282], each participant checked to have had Facebook and Telegram accounts and then registered the groups into two groups clustered by the distance on geographical location. These two groups are the intervention receiving group (group A) and the control group (group B) (**Figure 3.4).**

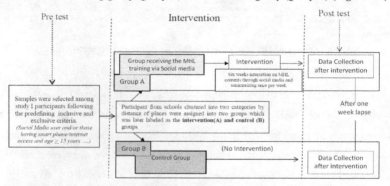

Figure 3.4: Study Roadmap and Procedures for the Intervention Study

For the intervention group, the texts, figures, and case vignettes were posted on both social media platforms every 72 hours on working days (every Monday and Thursday), for an approximate total of eight sessions spanning approximately six weeks in a row. After each week's sessions and every other session, there were discussion and summary sessions. The control group received information on academic advice titled secrets of successful students at the same frequency and on the same timescale as the other groups. At the end of week seven-one week after the conclusion of the intervention, post-test data collection was carried out from all of the participants in the study (i.e., both the intervention group and the control group).

To improve recruitment, compliance, and retention rates among study participants, we offered each participant a 45-megabyte internet package. Potential effect modifiers, confounding factors, and strict eligibility criteria were employed to maintain control over bias. A data clerk double-checked all data entries.

3.3.5. Variables and Measurement Tools

The socio-demographic variables used for this part of the thesis were gender, school grade, and age. The mental health literacy score was the primary study outcome variable. Primary independent variables were whether adolescents were assigned to the intervention group ($G_i=1$) or the control group ($G_i=0$) and whether they were given a pretest (t=0) or a post-test (t=1). The intervention implementation outcome measures and influencing factors were other study variables. The health literacy questionnaire [258], a freely available and validated instrument used in adolescent populations[262], was used to measure mental health literacy. In the context of the present investigation, we determined that the questionnaire was reliable (Cronbach's alpha = 0.834). The version of the MHLQ that was used in this investigation contained 33 questions. Based on a Likert scale, respondents responded to each question that ranged from 1 (strongly disagree) to 5 (strongly agree). Strongly disagreeing is indicated by 1, slightly disagreeing by 2, unsure about neither agreeing nor disagreeing is indicated by 3, unsure about neither agreeing nor disagreeing is indicated by 4, and strongly agreeing by 5. Statements regarding awareness, knowledge, attitudes, and beliefs regarding mental health issues were included in the survey[17,20–23].

The second aim of this part of the thesis was to investigate the contents of outcome measures associated with intervention implementation (acceptability, appropriateness, and feasibility)[117],[208]. An adapted version of a satisfaction questionnaire about social media health interventions (CSQ-I) was included[118].

Adolescents' viewpoints on the acceptability, appropriateness, and feasibility of the intervention's implementation and their level of satisfaction with the intervention were measured using these questionnaires. These questionnaire items elicited a response using a Likert scale with five points, each representing a different level of agreement: 1 = completely disagree, 2 = disagree, 3 = neither agree nor disagree, 4 = agree, and 5=completely agree. The intervention's acceptability, feasibility, appropriateness, and satisfaction were evaluated with the help of outcome measures to determine the degree to which each factor was met.

The participants were asked about the degree to which they liked the intervention, whether or not they found it appealing, and whether or not they found it welcoming. These four questions were used to determine whether or not the intervention was acceptable to the participants. The feasibility of the intervention approach was evaluated based on how easily it could be carried out, if it was even feasible at all, how straightforward it would be to apply, and so on. Four indicators of appropriateness were used to evaluate whether the intervention process seemed to fit its purpose, whether or not it was suitable, whether or not it was applicable, and whether or not it was a good match. The participants rated the quality of the intervention, whether or not it was wanted, whether or not it met the participant's needs, whether or not it was recommendable to others, the extent to which it helped them deal with their problems, and the extent to which they would like to repeat the experience. Satisfaction was measured using a seven-item questionnaire. Satisfaction was measured by rating the quality of the intervention.

A Likert scale with five points was used to measure the factors that were anticipated to influence the effectiveness of the intervention and the implementation outcome measures. Participants were asked to indicate their experience of personal and family-related challenges, as well as their level of perceived access to resources. These aspects could have been accounted for in the analyses if desired.

The anticipated factors influencing the intervention's effectiveness and implementation outcome measures were measured using a 5-point Likert scale. Participants were asked to indicate their perceived level of access to resources and their experience of personal and family-related challenges. These factors could be controlled for in the analyses.

3.3.6. Statistical Analyses

The descriptive statistics of the socio-demographic characteristics were utilized in the firsthand analysis. After that, the intervention effectiveness was evaluated by calculating the effect size and the difference-in-differences estimate. In the end, an investigation into the implementation outcome measures and the associated influencing factors was carried out. SPSS version 25 was utilized for each statistical analysis[283].

3.3.6.1. Effectiveness of the Intervention

Steven's measurement framework was followed[284]. The scores on the mental health literacy assessment were interpreted as intervals. When individuals' scores were computed, the negatively keyed items of the mental health literacy questionnaire (Q7, Q12, Q15, Q17, Q24, and Q26) were scored in reverse, ensuring consistency with positively keyed terms. Because of potential selection bias and other factors that could cloud the results, the study was limited to specific subsets of groups and characteristics. We first estimated the magnitude of the effect by computing the mean differences (the difference between the posttest and the pretest score) for each group using a paired t-test. The effectiveness of the intervention program was demonstrated and assessed using effect size and difference-in-differences calculations, and it was taken as significant at $p \leq 0.05$.

3.3.6.1.1. Effect Size Analysis

As stated by the recommendations of Jacob Cohen[114,285], the effect size is typically thought of as the most important outcome measure in studies that investigate practical interventions and the impacts of those interventions. In evidence-based and field-based studies of interventions, the effect size is the preferred method for communicating the practical significance of a result[286,287]. It was estimated using a 95% confidence interval, and its value was expressed using Cohen's d and Hedges' g. These expressions use a pooled standard deviation in the denominator, but the latter expression uses n while the former uses n-1. Both of these approaches to calculating the standard deviation represent the difference in the mean score between the intervention group and the control group. As a result, the absolute effect size is defined as the difference in the mental health literacy score between these two groups. Both the conventional and comparison methods were utilized to decipher the significance of this intervention's effect. The conventional method utilized a comprehensive point of reference, while the comparison method relied on prior research to decipher the meaning[114,115].

3.3.6.1.2. Difference-in-differences Analysis

Analysis of difference-in-differences was another method utilized to determine how effective the intervention was at improving mental health literacy (**Figure 3.5**). The difference-in-differences(DID) analysis is a type of regression analysis that investigates the data's time dimension to define the intervention's actual effect due to the intervention as well as the counterfactual effect effects of the intervention[116]. It was determined by analyzing the disparity in outcomes between the intervention and control groups throughout the intervention period, which lasted six weeks.

The disparity before the intervention program's implementation was estimated by analyzing the presence of unobserved heterogeneity[116]. A method of analysis like this has benefits when it comes to controlling for differences caused by unobservable characteristics. As a result, the intervention effect was obtained by determining the difference between the groups, as demonstrated in **Figure 3.5** illustrates the procedures utilized during the analysis. After computing the difference between before and after for each group [$E(YI_{ai}-YI_{bi}|D_i=1)$ and $E(YC_{ai}-YC_{bi}|D_i=0)$], the average intervention effect was computed [$E(YI_{ai}-YI_{bi}|D_i=1)-E(YC_{ai}-YC_{bi}|D_i=0)$, where the subscript a denotes "after," and b represents "before" the intervention. The intervention group is denoted by superscript I, and the control group is denoted by superscript C. If unit g is subjected to the intervention during period t, then D_{gt} is equal to 1, but it is equal to 0 if unit g is subjected to the control condition during period t. The outcome of interest for unit g during period t is denoted by the variable $Y(1)_{gt}$. This is the case in the hypothetical scenario in which unit g received the treatment during the period t. Under the alternative scenario, where g was assigned the control condition, the same unit and time result is denoted by the letter $Y(0)_{gt}$.

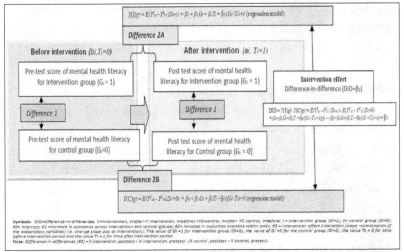

Figure 3. 5: Conceptual framework, regression model, and coefficients for the estimation of the difference-in-differences effect

Certain assumptions are used to calculate the difference-in-differences regression estimate[116]. The unobserved heterogeneity is assumed to be consistent over time, and this assumption is tested by contrasting the initial state with the final one. According to the common trend assumption, when intervention or treatment is not present, the control and intervention groups experience the same measurement trend of outcome variables over time. This is true even if the intervention or treatment is changed. Therefore, any deviation from the trend observed in the intervention group could be attributed to the effect of the intervention. In addition, it was assumed that all relationships are linear, that observations are independent, that there is no perfect collinearity, that the variances of the independent variables are not zero, and that error terms are normally distributed and have a value of zero. All of these assumptions were taken into consideration during this analysis.

It is presumed that if there had been no intervention, the difference between the "intervention" and "control" groups would have remained the same over time. The two groups would have developed the same way if there had been no intervention. As a result, the standard deviation of the outcomes for the control group is $\beta0$ during the pre-intervention time and $\beta0+\beta2$ during the post-intervention time. Similarly, the average untreated result in the intervention group during the pre-intervention time is $\beta0+\beta1$, and the average untreated result during the post-treatment period is $\beta0 + \beta1 +$

$\beta2$, where $\beta1$ is different regardless of the effect of the intervention. As a result, the difference in the pre-test should be assumed and anticipated. In contrast, the post-test difference can result from a causal effect (difference-in-differences, $\beta3$).

These assumptions narrow the field of potential confounding factors in the difference-in-differences analysis by focusing on factors not wholly determined by the random assignment. It was assumed that the confounders that vary across the groups do not change over time and that the confounders that do change over time remain the same. Because of this, the difference-in-difference is estimated with the help of a model that considers measures of the target variable, group membership, and periods. An estimate of the treatment effect can be obtained by examining the interaction term coefficient ($\beta3$). Notably, the timing effect is not the same in the intervention group as in the control group. The two groups start distinct, and the observable characteristics continue to shift over time.

3.3.6.2. Implementation Outcome Measures and the Influencing Factors

Descriptive analyses were used for each of the respective outcome measures and the response on the level of agreement. The mean score and differences ($p \leq 0.05$) across gender, age groups, and school grades were analyzed using an independent t-test scale of 1–5, with a value of 5 corresponding to the highest level of acceptability, appropriateness, feasibility, and satisfaction. Similarly, a descriptive analysis was used for each score of the respective factors that were anticipated to influence measures of the implementation outcomes and the potential effectiveness of the intervention program.

3.4. Ethical Consideration

The study has complied with regulations of the International Ethical Guidelines for Health-Related Research Involving Humans[288]. Ethical approval was obtained from the KIIT University, KIMS, Institutional Ethics committee *(Reference: KIIT/KIMS/IEC/63/2019)* and Haramaya University, College of Health and Medical Sciences Institutional Health Research Review Ethics Committee *(Reference: 00. H.M.S./10.0/3763/2020.* Written informed consent was obtained from all participants. The parents of adolescents for a child under fifteen years had offered their consent, and adolescents of fifteen and above years were factored out following the school counselors and school principals' adequate explanation about their level of maturity and decisional capacity with due reference to the guideline[288]. However, as duly authorized representatives, respective school principals had expressed their consent both orally and signed on consent forms for all participants. Participants had the right to ask for information about the study anytime and unhindered the right not to participate. The response of the participants remained confidential.

Chapter Summary

The thesis has consisted of two consecutive study designs: cross-sectional and quasi-experimental (intervention effectiveness). The study design and analysis for both studies are quantitative. It was conducted in Dire Dawa, Ethiopia, among adolescents attending schooling.

A multistage and random sampling strategy was used to contact 934 adolescents in grades 5 through 12 at public and private schools. About 731 responded with an 80.10% response rate. Preexisting and validated mental health literacy (MHL) questionnaire, the strength and difficulty questionnaire (SDQ), and the WHO-5 well-being index were used for data collection. SPSS version 25 was used for statistical analysis. The statistical analysis involved descriptive statistics, variance (ANOVA) analysis with one direction, and a hierarchical multivariable linear regression analysis. The prevalence of mental conditions (caseness) was decomposed into normal (80 %), borderline (80-90 %), and abnormal (>90 %) categories using the original three-band categorization, which used cut-off scores just at 80th and 90th percentile. The correlation analysis was employed to evaluate the association between the strength difficulties scale scores and adolescent mental health literacy scores. The prevalence of perceived mental health issues and effects of socio-demographic factors were estimated. The impact of socio-demographic characteristics was reported in terms of the odds ratio for each category using a confidence interval of 95% ($p<0.05$). A score p-value of less than or equal to 0.05 was used as the baseline for determining statistical significance at a calculated 95% confidence interval.

The quasi-experimental study was employed to investigate the difference in change in mental health literacy scores of the intervention (treatment) and control groups. Six weeks were allocated to the presentation of the mental health literacy program. The data were gathered after the intervention from both the intervention (treatment) and control groups. Effect size and difference-in-differences model were carried out with a confidence interval of 95% and $p \leq 0.05$.

CHAPTER FOUR

RESULTS

CHAPTER FOUR
4. RESULTS

4.1. Brief on the Findings of the Thesis

The result section of the thesis is organized into the order of objectives. The presentation of findings for the part I of the thesis (cross-sectional) is followed by part II of the thesis (intervention). The cross-sectional(part-I) of the thesis includes (i) socio-demographic characteristics, (ii) mental health literacy level, (iii) the relationship between mental health literacy and socio-demographic characteristics, (iv) self–reported mental health issues, the associated socio-demographic factors and (v) the correlation of self–reported mental health issues and mental health literacy among school adolescents in an urban Ethiopia are reported. In the second part of the study (part-II), the effect size and difference-in-difference analysis have been demonstrated to examine the intervention program's effectiveness and success in improving adolescents' mental health literacy. Within this section of the report, the secondary analysis explored the four measures of the outcomes of the intervention's implementation: the acceptability of the implementation, the appropriateness of the implementation, the feasibility of the implementation, and the satisfaction of the beneficiaries. In addition, the perceived factors that affect the effectiveness of the intervention and these outcome measures are reported. Hence, the findings are presented in the following order as outlined below.

⊥ **Findings for part-I of the thesis (cross-sectional study)**
  ➤ Socio-demographic characteristics
  ➤ Level of adolescent mental health literacy
  ➤ The effect of socio-demographic factors on mental health literacy
  ➤ The cut-point for self-completed SDQ score with a baseline reference
  ➤ Strength difficulty scores and perceived mental health issues
  ➤ Association of mental health issues and socio-demographic factors
  ➤ Correlation of mental health literacy with strength difficulty scores and well-being index

⬦ **Findings for part II of the thesis (Intervention Study)**
  ➤ Socio-demographic characteristics
  ➤ Mental health literacy pre-and post-
  ➤ Effect of the intervention on the mental health literacy of adolescents
      o Effect size estimate of the intervention
      o Difference-in-difference estimates of the intervention
  ➤ Implementation outcome measures and influencing factors
      o Implementation Outcome Measures
      o Perceived influencing factors

4.2. Findings for part-I of the Thesis (Cross-sectional Study)

4.2.1. Socio-demographic Characteristics

From the approached 934 potential participants, 751(80.41%) filled the questionnaire, and 20 respondents were removed from the analysis due to having significant missing data. The Socio-demographic characteristics of these study participants are presented in **Table 4.1**.

Table 4. 1: Socio-demographic characteristics of study participants

Socio-demographic Characteristics	Male (n=366)	Female (n=365)	P value
Mean age (SD*)	16.27(2.19)	15.95(2.02)	0.037
Age group years			
Ethnicity / Cultural affiliation			
Amhara	20.5%	29.9%	≤ .001
Oromo	30.0%	19.5%	
Somali	24.4%	25.7%	
Others	25.1%	24.9%	
Age group in years			
11-13	13.7%	12.9%	.079
14-16	36.6%	44.6%	
17-19	49.7%	42.5%	
School grade level			
Upper elementary Grade 5-8	39.3%	43.0%	.571
Lower Secondary Grade 9-10	39.6%	40.0%	
Upper secondary Grade 11-12	21.1%	17.0%	
Maternal education level			
Non-educated	63.7%	60.5%	.575
Elementary Level	8.5%	9.3%	
Secondary level	19.9%	23.6%	
College or above	7.9%	6.6%	
Paternal education level			
Non-educated	54.6%	54.2%	.128
Elementary Level	5.7%	2.5%	
Secondary level	24.6%	28.2%	
College or above	15.1%	15.1%	

4.2.2. Level of Adolescent Mental Health Literacy

The mean score of mental health literacy was normally distributed (Skewness=-1.321, Kurtosis=2.804) with a mean of 135.98 and SD=15.50; these scores were affected by socio-demographic characteristics. Males had slightly lower levels of mental health literacy (133.84) than females (138.12) (p<0.01). Regarding the formal normality test, skewness and kurtosis of the distribution are preferable over the eyeball test for both small and large samples. The formal normality tests (skewness and kurtosis) were preferred over the eyeball test to evaluate the normality of the data distribution. An asymmetric distribution is said to have skewness, while a peak distribution is said to have kurtosis. We use a skewness absolute value of less than two or a kurtosis absolute value of less than 7 for determining the substantial normality that the present findings fulfilled[278]. Hence, the mental health literacy score presented by graphs showed an absolute skew value far less than two and the absolute kurtosis (proper) far less than seven. According to findings illustrated in **Figure 4.1**, gender differed significantly in participants' levels of mental health literacy, with female participants demonstrating a slightly higher level of mental health literacy(M=138.12, SD=13.588) than male participants(M=133.64, SD=16.945), F(1,729)=6.120, p=0.014.

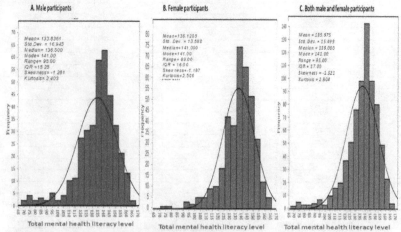

Figure 4.1: Descriptive analysis of mental health literacy for (a) male, (b) female, and (c) both male and female participants.

4.2.3. The Effect of Socio-demographic Factors on Mental Health Literacy

Adolescents had different levels of mental health literacy across different ethnic groups and cultural affiliations, which was true for both male and female adolescents. It was significantly different between male adolescents of different ethnic and cultural affiliations, with mental health literacy scores of Amhara (M=135.83, SD=16.93), Oromo (M=133.59, SD=15.71), Somalia (M=124.48, SD=18.03), and other ethnic and cultural affiliations(M=138.90, SD=16.08), $(F(3,362)=6.115, p\leq0.01)$. Among female adolescents, mental health literacy scores were significantly different who were identified as Amhara (M=140.56, SD=12.96), Oromo(M=134.74, SD=15.11), Somalia (M=132.24, SD=12.37), and other ethnic/cultural affiliations (M=135.44, SD=9.71), $(F(3,361)=7.243, p \leq0.01)$.

The maternal education level $(F(3,361)=2.866, p=0.037)$ and the grade level of the adolescents$(F(2,362)=4.466, p=0.012)$ were significantly associated with the mental health literacy of the adolescent females. However, the educational level of the male adolescent parents was not significantly associated with the male adolescent mental health literacy. There were no statistically significant effects of paternal education discovered for either the female $(F(3,362)=0.360, p= 0.782)$ or the male $(F(2,363) =1.811, p = 0.165)$ participants in this study (**Table 4.2**).

Table 4.2: The effect of socio-demographic characteristics on mental health literacy (One-way ANOVA at p<0.05, 95% CI)

Socio-demographic characteristics	Mental health literacy level					
	Male adolescents			Female adolescents		
	Mean score(SD)	95% CI	p-value	Mean score(SD)	95% CI	p-value
Total (altogether)	133.84(16.95)	132.09-135.58		138.12(13.59)	136.72-139.52	
Ethnicity/cultural affiliation						
Amhara	135.83(16.93)	133.28-138.37	≤.001	140.56(12.96)	138.87-142.25	≤.001
Oromo	133.59(15.71)	130.87-136.32		134.74(15.11)	131.31-138.17	
Somali	124.48(18.03)	119.00-129.96		132.24(12.37)	128.38-136.09	
Others	138.90(16.08)	131.38-146.42		135.44(9.71)	130.61-140.28	
School grade						
Grade 5-8	135.01(14.70)	132.59-137.43	.165	138.57(13.26)	136.48-140.66	.012
Grade 9-10	131.77(18.83)	128.68-134.86		135.99(14.65)	133.60-138.39	
Grade 11-12	135.52(16.94)	131.67-139.36		141.98(10.74)	139.26-144.71	
Maternal education						
Non-educated	132.72(16.60)	130.58-134.86	.054	137.01(13.22)	135.26-138.76	.037
Elementary	131.94(19.51)	124.78-139.09		137.85(12.77)	133.40-142.31	
Secondary	138.71(13.79)	135.49-141.93		141.77(14.20)	138.72-144.81	
College	132.55(22.04)	124.17-140.94		135.67(14.23)	129.66-141.68	
Paternal education						
Non-educated	133.20(16.86)	130.85-135.55	.7820	138.24(12.50)	136.49-139.99	.844
Elementary	134.95(14.79)	128.22-141.68		134.67(17.23)	121.43-147.91	
Secondary	133.81(17.14)	130.22-137.40		137.79(15.89)	134.68-140.89	
College	135.76(17.96)	130.91-140.62		138.87(12.28)	135.55-142.19	

The level of respondents' mental health literacy negatively correlated with their age for both male and female respondents (**Table 4.3**). Ethnicity also had a significant association with mental health literacy. Adolescents who were Somali, Oromo, and other ethnic groups or cultural affiliations($p \leq 0.01$) exhibited lower mental health literacy than those with an Amhara ethnic/cultural affiliation. There was a correlation between the level of mental health literacy and school grade, and this finding was especially significant for the female respondents ($p \leq 0.01$). The effect of the education level of the mother and the father had a different bearing on male and female participants(**Table 4.3**).

Table 4.3: Socio-demographic factors associated with mental health literacy among male and female adolescents (bi-variate analysis adjusting for age showing coefficient at (p≤0.05, 95% CI)

Socio-demographic factors	Male Coefficient (95%CI)	Female Coefficient (95%CI)
Age (years)	-0.511(-1.307-0.285)	-.425(-1.117-.267)
Ethnicity/cultural affiliation		
Amhara (Ref.)		
Oromo	-3.682(-7.493-.130)**	-6.170(-9.586-(-2.753)**
Somali	-12.968(-18.377-(-7.560)**	-8.638(-12.931-(-4.346)**
Others	-5.828(-13.355-1.699)	-5.281(-11.894-1.332)
School grade		
Grade 11-12 (Ref.)		
Grade 9-10	-2.621(-7.138-1.896)	-6.190(-10.021-(-2.359)**
Grade 5-8	-.86(-5.527-3.797)	-3.645(-7.520-.230)
Maternal education		
College (Ref.)		
secondary education	1.926(-5.662-9.514)	5.885(-.357-12.127)
elementary education	-3.661(-12.417-5.094)	2.581(-4.562-9.723)
non- educated	-2.262(-9.131-4.606)	1.311(-4.507-7.128)
Paternal education		
College (Ref.)		
secondary education	1.096(-4.653-6.845)	-1.854(-6.337-2.629)
elementary education	2.898(-5.561-11.356)	-3.997(-13.520-5.526)
non-education	1.442(-3.666-6.550)	-.882(-4.946-3.182)

** $P<0.001$,   * $P<0.01$

The contribution of socio-demographic variables to explaining the variations in mental health literacy was revealed by multiple regression analysis **(Table 4.4)**. Cultural and ethnic affiliation explained the most variation (6.3% in females and 6.1% in males) in mental health literacy. Grade/education level minimally accounted for variability among males (0.8%) and females (2.5%). The analysis was done by coding either father or mother education level as one variable for the regression model, unlike analysis done separately for ANOVA. About 2.0% of adolescents' mental health literacy variance was accounted for by mothers' and fathers' education levels. Parents' education level was independently associated with the mental health literacy of adolescents and negatively associated with the respondents' grades in school. When taken together, 10.7% variance in the mental health literacy of female adolescents and 8.9% of the variability in the mental health literacy of male adolescents accounted for these factors **(Table 4.4)**.

Table 4.4: Socio-demographic factors associated with mental health literacy level among male and female adolescents in an Urban Ethiopia (Hierarchical multivariate linear regression analysis showing coefficient and 95% CI).

Socio-demographic characteristics	Male Adolescents						Female Adolescents					
	Model 1		Model 2		Model 3		Model 1		Model 2		Model 3	
	Coeff	95%CI	Coeff	95% CI	Coeff	95% CI	Coeff	95%CI	Coeff	95%CI	Coeff	95%CI
Ethnicity/cultural affiliation												
Amhara(Ref.)												
Oromo	-3.682	-7.493,0.130	-3.082	-7.150,.985	-3.214	-7.423,.996	-6.17	-9.586,-2.753	-5.213	-8.701,-1.725	-5.243	-8.912,-1.575
Somali	-12.968	-18.377,-7.560**	-14.315	-19.987,-8.643	-14.569	-20.405,-8.733	-8.638	-12.931,-4.346	-9.569	-13.971,-5.168	-8.968	-13.465,-4.471
Others	-5.828	-13.355,1.699	-5.092	-12.657,2.473	-4.687	-12.296,2.921	-5.281	-13.226,-2.754	-4.962	-13.106,-4.653	-4.668	-13.29,-3.765
School grade												
Grade 11-12(Ref.)												
Grade 9-10			-3.945	-8.666,.777	-3.658	-8.447,1.131			-5.872	-9.716,-2.028	-5.898	-9.795,-2.000
Grade 5-8			-4.316	-9.114,.482	-4.267	-9.113,.578			-5.13	-9.038,-1.222	-4.941	-8.923,-.959
Parental (father and/or mother) education												
College (Ref.)												
Secondary education					3.356	-2.583,9.295					-1.69	-9.83,5.83
Elementary education					8.248	-.711,17.208					-0.297	-19.753,9.543
Non-education					6.797	.872,12.723					1.276	-9.792,6.345
R²	0.061		0.069		0.089		0.063		0.087		0.107	
Adjusted R²			0.056		0.058				0.074		0.076	
ΔR²			0.01		0.02				0.024		0.021	
F (p value)	<0.001		0.165		0.363		≤0.001		0.009		0.362	

Notes: *Factors included in the models: Model 1: Ethnic/cultural affiliation; Model 2: Model 1+ school grade of the adolescents; Model 3: Model 2+ Parental education status. ** P<0.001,   * P<0.01, Coeff = Coefficients*

4.2.4. The Cut-point for Self-completed SDQ Score with a Baseline Reference

Under this subheading, the cut-off point for self-completed SDQ score with baseline reference ranges (caseness for mental health issues), the effect of socio-demographic characteristics, and the correlation of self–reported mental health issues and mental health literacy among school adolescents were presented. The original 3 band (cut-off scores at 80th & 90th) was used to determine and estimate adolescents' perceived mental health issues. The newer 4 band (cut-off scores at 80th, 90th & 95th) categorizations are reported for comparison (Table 4.5)

Table 4.5: The cut of scores for baseline reference ranges (caseness) for both the original 3 band and the newer 4 band categorization

Self-completed SDQ	Original 3 band categories(cut-off scores at 80th & 90th)						Newer 4 band categorisations (cut-off scores at 80th, 90th & 95th)							
	Normal		Borderline		Abnormal		Close to average		Slightly raised slightly lowered		High (/low)		Very high (very low)	
	Baseline norm	Present study range	Baseline norm	Present study range	Baseline norm	Present study range	Baseline norm	Present study range	Baseline norm	Present study range	Baseline norm	Present study range	Baseline norm	Present study range
Total difficulties score	0-15	0-14	16-19	15-17	20-40	18-40	0-14	0-14	15-17	15-17	18-19	18-20	20-40	20-40
Emotional problems score	0-5	0-5	6	6	7-10	7-10	0-4	0-5	5	6	6	7	7-10	8-10
Conduct problems score	0-3	0-3	4	4	5-10	5-10	0-3	0-3	4	4	5	5	6-10	6-10
Hyperactivity score	0-5	0-4	6	5	7-10	6-10	0-5	0-4	6	5	7	6	8-10	7-9
Peer problems score	0-3	0-4	4-5	5	6-10	6-10	0-2	0-4	3	5	4	6	5-10	7-9
Pro-social score	6-10	6-10	5	5	0-4	0-4	7-10	7-10	6	6	5	5	0-4	0-4
Externalising score	0-5	0-5	6-10	6-7	11-20	8-20	0-5	0-5	6-10	6-7	11-12	8	13-20	9-20
Internalising score	0-4	0-8	5-8	9-10	9-20	11-20	0-4	0-8	5-8	9-10	9-10	11-12	11-20	13-20

4.2.5. Strength Difficulty Scores and Perceived Mental Health Issues

The participants' total difficulty and subscale scores were shown across gender and school grade (**Figure 4.2**). The externalization and internalizing problems presented with the corresponding difficulty subscale scores gender and grade levels (**Figure 4.3**).

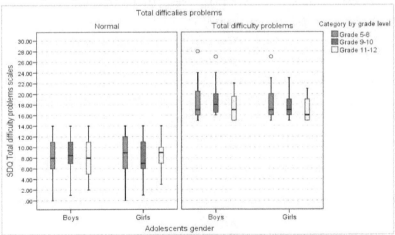

Figure 4.2: Self-completed total strength and difficulty score with total difficulty problems across gender and grade level compared to the normal

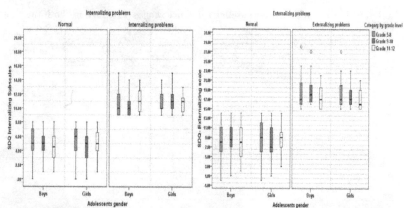

Figure 4.3: Internalizing and externalizing difficulties are indicated using self-completed strength difficulty subscale scores across gender and grade level.

These mental health issues expressed with the total difficulties and subscales were higher for female adolescents than male adolescents. The school adolescent's mental health problems (cases from total difficulties and subscales) were presented across gender and age categories (**Figure 4.4**). Prevalence of mental health problems (total difficulties, internalizing, emotional and peer relationship problems) were higher viz. total difficulties (15.9-25.5%), internalizing (14.9-28.4%), emotional (10.4-23.9%), and peer relationship (17.8-25.8%) problems. The prevalence of mental health problems subscales was greater than 20% for female and male adolescents. The most common mental health issue is depression, often measured by the well-being index (WHO-5) per the depression (ICD-10) inventory. A raw score of less than 13 or a score of 0 or 1 on any five items on the well-being index (WHO-5) is the cut-off score for depression(ICD-10). It was higher (25.5%) for female adolescents within 14-16 years.

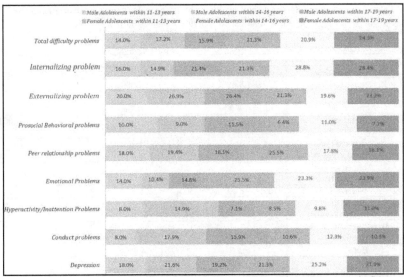

Figure 4.4: Prevalence of mental health problems among school adolescents in Dire Dawa, Ethiopia.

4.2.6. Association of Mental Health Issues and Socio-demographic Factors

Statistical difference in prevalence was examined for each banding of subscale (Chi-square test) as per the original-3 band categorization (cut-off scores at 80th & 90th) between males and females (**Table 4.6**). It was found that the proportion of abnormal females with total difficulties and emotional and internalizing problems was higher than males ($p<0.05$). The prevalence of conduct and externalizing problems was highly associated with being male than female.

Table 4.6: Chi-square test of mental health problems prevalence as per the original 3 band categorization (cut-off scores at 80th & 90th) between males and females

Sub-scales and bandings	Males (n=366)		Females (n=365)		df	X^2	p
	n	%	n	%			
Total difficulties					2	6.913ª	0.042
Normal(0-14)	307	83.9%	283	77.5%			
Borderline(15-17)	29	7.9%	48	13.2%			
Abnormal(18-40)	30	8.2%	34	9.3%			
Emotional problems score					2	14.442 ª	0.001
Normal0-5)	318	86.9%	278	76.2%			
Borderline=6	23	6.3%	36	9.9%			
Abnormal(7-10)	25	6.8%	51	14.0%			
Conduct problems							
Normal(0-3)	309	84.4%	324	88.8%	2	3.674ª	0.159
Borderline=4	30	8.2%	18	4.9%			
Abnormal(5-10)	25.0	7.4%	25.0	6.3%			
Hyperactivity score					2	0.488ª	0.783
Normal (0-4)	329	89.9%	328	89.9%			
Borderline=5	21	5.7%	18	4.9%			
Abnormal(6-10)	16	4.4%	19	5.2%			
Peer problems score					2	0.930ª	0.628
Normal(0-4)	298	81.4%	296	81.1%			
Borderline=5	41	11.2%	36	9.9%			
Abnormal(6-10)	27	7.4%	33	9.0%			
Internalizing score					2	9.332ª	0.009
Normal(0-8)	299	81.7%	264	72.3%			
Borderline(9-10)	36	9.8%	50	13.7%			
Abnormal(11-20)	31	8.5%	51	14.0%			
Externalizing score					2	1.896ª	0.387
Normal(0-5)	272	74.3%	287	78.6%			
Borderline(6-7)	50	13.7%	41	11.2%			
Abnormal(8-20)	44	12.0%	37	10.1%			
Pro-social score					2	0.549ª	0.760
Normal(6-10)	328	89.6%	332	91.0%			
Borderline=5	18	4.9%	14	3.8%			
Abnormal(0-4)	20	5.5%	19	5.2%			

The effect of socio-demographic characteristics on mental health issues was analyzed using binary logistic regression (**Table 4.7**). Binary logistic regression analysis showed that mental health problems odds were significantly associated with some socio-demographic characteristics (p<0.05). Females had reportedly a substantially higher prevalence of mental health problems in upper elementary (AOR: 2.60 (0.95-7.10)) and lower secondary levels (AOR: 2.73 (1.19-6.29) compared to upper secondary grade level (p<0.05); but it was not significantly different for males. It was twice higher among adolescents with a self and family members experiencing psychoactive substances use (p<0.05). Prevalence difference across age, maternal and paternal education, and employment status was insignificant (p>0.05).

However, the prevalence was not significantly different for males by education level. Prevalence difference was insignificant across the three age groups, maternal and paternal education level, and types of jobs or level of employment (p>0.05). Adolescents who experienced psychoactive substance use themselves or their family members were more likely to suffer mental health problems (p<0.05). Differences in prevalence existed but were insignificant across the three age groups, maternal and paternal education level, and types of jobs or level of employment (p>0.05).

Table 4.7: Association of mental health problems and socio-demographic determinants analyzed with binary logistic regression

Predictors	Categories	Male		Female	
		UAOR(95% CI)	AOR(95% CI)	UAOR(95% CI)	AOR(95% CI)
Age group(years)	11-19	-	-	-	-
	11-13	1	1	1	1
	14-16	1.27(0.51-3.18)	0.959(0.25-3.7)	0.98 (0.44-2.16)	0.65 (0.20-2.06)
	17-19	1.16(0.48-2.84)	0.643(0.06-6.28)	1.20 (0.55-2.64)	0.53 (0.08-3.38)
Grade level	Upper elementary (5-8)	1.08(0.51-2.31)	1.44(0.50-4.15)	1.57 (0.70-3.50)	2.60 (0.95-7.10)
	Lower Secondary (9-10)	1.02(0.48-2.18)	1.11(0.50-2.46)	2.22 (1.00-4.92)*	2.73 (1.19-6.29)*
	Upper secondary (11-12)	1	1	1	1
Experience with Psychoactive substances use					
Self-experience	No	1	1	1	1
	Yes	0.45(0.22-0.93)*	2.20(1.07-4.52)*	2.17 (0.95-4.95)	2.16 (0.95-4.92)
Any Family Experience	No	1	1	1	1
	Yes	2.01(1.01-4.00)*	2.04(1.01-4.09)*	1.07(0.63-1.84)	1.06 (0.62-1.81)
Parents practicing corporal punishment	No	1	1	1	1
	Yes	1.24 (0.69-2.24)	1.24 (0.69-2.23)	1.43 (0.82-2.51)	1.33 (0.75-2.36)
Adolescents report	No	1	1	1	1
Perceived worry about family problems	Yes	1.186(0.64-2.21)	1.17(0.62-2.20)	1.24 (0.73-2.12)	1.20 (0.70-2.06)
Mother education level	Non-educated	1	1	1	1
	Elementary	1.31(0.50-3.43)	1.30 (0.49-3.41)	1.99 (0.57-6.96)	0.73 (0.29-1.87)
	Secondary	1.30(0.66-2.57)	1.30 (0.66-2.58)	1.50 (0.34-6.70)	1.37 (0.78-2.42)
	College or above	0.63(0.18-2.20)	0.64 (0.18-2.24)	2.71 (0.74-9.93)	0.52 (0.15-1.81)
Father education level	Non-educated	1	1	1	1
	Elementary	1.51 (0.47-4.82)	1.48 (0.46-4.74)	1.03 (0.21-5.14)	1.00 (0.20-4.99)
	Secondary	1.60 (0.83-3.09)	1.61 (0.83-3.11)	1.04 (0.58-1.84)	1.07 (0.60-1.90)
	college or above	1.42 (0.64-3.16)	1.45 (0.65-3.23)	1.23 (0.61-2.46)	1.20 (0.60-2.41)
Mother job	Housewife/Unemployed	1	1	1	1
	Work in private	0.79 (0.41-1.51)	0.79 (0.41-1.51)	1.40 (0.77-2.53)	1.40 (0.77-2.54)
	Employed	0.44 (0.16-1.22)	0.44 (0.16-1.21)	0.55 (0.22-1.42)	0.55 (0.21-1.44)
Father job	Unemployed/Jobless	1	1	1	1
	Work in private	1.24 (0.66-2.32)	1.24 (0.66-2.33)	0.75(0.43-1.33)	0.77(0.44-1.36)
	Employed	2.56 (0.75-8.74)	2.52 (0.73-8.70)	ns	ns

** Significant at p<0.01   * Significant at p<0.05

~ 92 ~

4.2.7. Correlation of Mental Health Literacy with Strength Difficulty Scores and Well-being Index

The bivariate correlations showed that the mental health literacy score was negatively associated with total strength difficulty score and subscale strength difficulties scores (emotional problems, peer problems, conduct problems, and hyperactivity-inattention) (Table 4.8).

Table 4. 8: Means, standard deviations, and correlations between mental health literacy, strength difficulties questionnaire scale, and subjective mental well-being

Variables	Measurement scale	Score range	Score	SD	Correlation coefficient (r)) with 95%CI		
					A	B	C
Mental well-being	WHO-5 scale (0-5)	0-25	16.39	5.83	1	-.319** (-.380-(-.253))	0.153** (.078-.233)
Total difficulties	SDQ Scale (0-25)	0-40	10.17	5.021	-.319** (-.380-(-.253))	1	-.114 (-.191-(-.038)
Mental health literacy	MHLQ33 Scale (1-5)	33-165	135.98	15.50	0.153** (.078-.233)	-.114** (-.191-(-.038))	1

**. Correlation is significant at the 0.01 level (2-tailed); *. Correlation is significant at the 0.05 level (2-tailed)

Table 4. 9: Correlations of strength difficulties score and subscales mean scores with mental health literacy score and subjective mental well-being

Variables	1	2	3	4	5	6	7	8	9
1. MHL Total mean Score	1	.160** (.084-.234)	-.135** (-.211-(-.064))	-.136** (-.212-(-.058))	-.006 (-.078-.058)	-.088* (-.165-(-.010))	-.166** (-.244-(-.087))	-.051 (-.120-.016)	-.124** (-.198-(-.052))
2. Mental wellbeing index		1	-.140** (-.206-(-.076))	-.281** (-.350-(-.210))	-.293** (-.366-(-.215))	-.130** (-.200-(-.060)	-.288** (-.329-(-.186))	-.279** (-.347-(-.209))	-.319** (-.388-(-.250))
3. SDQ Conduct problems subscale mean Score			1	.345** (.275-.412)	.228** (.159-.301)	.294** (.220-.368)	.812** (.785-.837)	.319** (.249-.388)	.652** (.607-.694)
4. SDQ Hyperactivity problems subscale mean Score				1	.385** (.310-.454)	.197** (.125-.265)	.828** (.802-.854)	.380** (.310-.446)	.700** (.656-.740)
5. SDQ Emotional problems subscale mean Score					1	.272** (.195-.342)	.376** (.301-.453)	.862** (.844-.880)	.749** (.714-.783)
6. SDQ Peer problems subscale mean Score						1	.298** (.231-.362)	.721** (.683-.756)	.617** (.570-.659)
7. SDQ Externalizing Problems subscale mean Score							1	.427** (.360-.489)	.825** (.798-.848)
8. SDQ Internalizing problems subscale mean Score								1	.863** (.842-.882)
9. SDQ Total difficulties problems Score									1

**. Correlation is significant at the 0.01 level (2-tailed); *. Correlation is significant at the 0.05 level (2-tailed)

4.3. Findings for part II of the Thesis (The Intervention Study)

4.3.1. Socio-demographic characteristics

Table 4.10 provides a demonstration of the socio-demographic characteristics of the participants. In the intervention group, the mean age of the participants was 17.34 years old with a standard deviation of 1.31 years, while in the control group, the mean age was 17.21 years old with a standard deviation of 1.36 years. There was no statistically significant difference between the groups in any demographic characteristics (i.e., all p>0.05).

Table 4.10: Summary of demographic characteristics for intervention and control groups

Demographic Characteristics		Intervention Group $(n_1=77)$	Control Group $(n_2=76)$	p -value
Mean Age		17.34±1.31	17.21±1.36	0.557
		n (%)	n (%)	
Sex	Boys	43 (55.84)	43 (56.68)	0.528
	Girls	34 (44.26)	33 (43.42)	
Age group (years)	15–17	34 (44.26)	35 (46.15)	0.471
	18–19	43 (55.84)	41 (53.95)	
Grade level	9–10	39 (50.65)	44 (57.89)	0.231
	11–12	38 (49.45)	32 (42.11)	

*Note: *Chi-square test.*

4.3.2. Mental health Literacy Pre-and Post-intervention

Participants' pretest and posttest mental health literacy scores in the intervention and control groups are presented by age and gender (**Figure 4.5**). Girls had slightly higher mean pretest and posttest mental health literacy scores than boys. The mean pretest and posttest mental health literacy scores in the control group were lower than in the intervention group. The paired-samples t-test revealed a statistically significant difference between mean pretest and posttest scores.

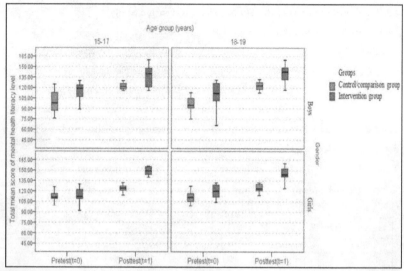

Figure4.5: The intervention and control groups' pretest and post-test mental health literacy scores.

4.3.3. Effectiveness of the Intervention on Mental Health Literacy of Adolescents

4.3.3.1. Effect Size Estimate of the Intervention

Analyses of paired samples with t-tests showed that the control and intervention groups showed a significant improvement in mental health literacy between the pre-test and post-test time points (p<0.01)(**Table 4.11**). However, the effect size estimates obtained from the intervention group were significantly larger than those obtained from the control group. The effect size for mental health literacy was most effective among young women between the ages of 15 and 17, particularly among teenage girls. Independent samples t-tests revealed that the intervention group had a significantly larger effect size than the control group (p<0.05). This effect size was found to be substantially more pronounced in females between the ages of 15 and 17 (Cohen's d=0.2.042, Hedges' g=2.045, p<0.01) than it was in males of the same age (Cohen's d=0.141, Hedges' g=0.141, p>0.05). In participants aged 18–19 years, the effect size was smaller than expected and failed to reach statistical significance (p>0.05) (**Table 4.11**).

Table 4.11: Effect size for total mental health literacy score in intervention and control groups by age and gender

Category		Intervention Group (n=77)		Control Group (n=76)		Effect Size			
		Total Mean Differences (Posttest-Pretest Score)	Confidence Interval 95%	Total Mean Differences (Posttest-Pretest Score)	Confidence Interval 95%	Cohen's d	Hedges' g	t-test	p-value
All	15–19	27.416	23.033–31.798	20.987	17.254–24.719	0.359	0.333	2.222	0.028
	15–17	26.879	20.377–33.381	19.139	13.280–24.998	0.445	0.438	1.848	0.069
	18–19	27.884	21.575–34.193	22.805	17.986–27.624	0.284	0.283	1.297	0.198
Boys	15–17	21.316	11.212–31.420	24.278	13.750–34.806	0.141	0.141	-0.428	0.672
	18–19	29.250	20.265–38.235	27.120	21.358–32.882	0.118	0.119	0.416	0.679
Girls	15–17	34.429	28.303–40.555	13.118	7.840–18.395	2.042	2.045	5.666	0.001
	18–19	26.158	16.562–35.754	16.063	7.978–24.147	0.570	0.564	1.661	0.106
Boys	15–19	25.744	19.201–32.289	25.930	20.646–31.214	0.012	0.012	-0.045	0.965
Girls	15–19	29.667	23.671–35.66	14.545	10.021–19.070	1.012	1.012	4.101	0.001

4.3.3.2. Difference-in-difference Estimates of the Intervention

Table 4.12 and **Figure 4.6** show a regression model stratified by sex, age group, and educational level for the difference-in-differences analysis. These models were used to estimate the results of the intervention. The intervention was evaluated to have a highly significant impact (DID: 0.348, CI: 0.154–0.542, p<0.001), supporting the proposed hypothesis. The increase in mental health literacy scores differed by sex and age.

Table 4. 12: Difference-in-Differences (DID) Estimating the Effect of the Intervention on the Mean Score of Mental Health Literacy

Category		DID Estimate	p-value	95% Confidence Interval DID Estimate
Sex	Altogether	0.348	<0.001	0.154–0.542
	Boys	0.308	<0.05	0.042–0.574
	Girls	0.398	<0.01	0.120–0.677
Age group	15–17 years	0.295	<0.05	0.020–0.570
	18–19 years	0.392	<0.001	0.117–0.667
School grade level	9–10	0.371	<0.01	0.096–0.646
	11–12	0.324	<0.05	0.050–0.597

Note: DID: estimates the mean of mental health literacy score change after controlling for (observable) confounders. **Abbreviations**: DID, difference-in-difference.

Table 4.12 demonstrated that the mental health literacy score was improved significantly despite differences associated with gender (DID for boys was 0.308, with a 95% confidence interval ranging from 0.042- 0.574, p<0.05, vs. DID for girls was 0.398, with a 95% confidence interval ranging from 0.120- 0.677, p< 0.01). The change in mean score of mental health literacy varied across age group and (15–17 years DID: 0.295, CI: 0.020–0.570, p<0.05 vs 18–19 DID: 0.392, CI: 0.117–0.667, p<0.001), and education level (grades 9–10 DID: 0.371, CI: 0.096–0.646, p <0.01 vs grades 11–12 DID: 0.324, CI: 0.050–0.597, p <0.05).

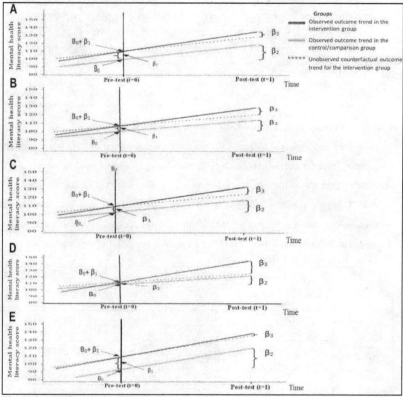

Figure 4.6: Difference-in-differences results of the intervention.
Note: The labels (A) for all participants, (B) males 15-17 years), (C) males 18-19 years, (D) females 15-17 years, and (E) females 18-19 years). Models were adjusted for age and education level.

4.3.4. Implementation Outcome Measures and Influencing Factors

These analyses aimed to evaluate the self-rated perceived implementation outcome measures and the potential factors that affect the effectiveness and implementation outcome measures.

4.3.4.1. Implementation Outcome Measures

Most respondents either 'completely agreed' or 'agreed' with the level of the intervention acceptability, feasibility, appropriateness, and satisfaction (**Figure 4.7**). Ratings varied significantly across age groups, with older adolescents reporting a higher proportion of complete agreement regarding acceptability, appropriateness, feasibility, and satisfaction. There was no significant correlation between ratings and gender (**Table 4.13**). More than sixty percent of those who took the survey provided responses indicating that they completely agreed with the acceptability of the implementation (range: fifty-five to seventy-two percent), the extent to which they liked it, found it appealing, and found its features welcoming. The ratings of its feasibility, which include how easily it can be implemented, carried out, accomplished, and utilized, ranged between 35 and 50 percent. Between 57 and 63 percent of respondents felt that the implementation was appropriate in terms of fitting, suitability, applicability, and the degree to which the implementation was a good match. The response to satisfaction score ranged from 45 to 71%, depending on the perceived quality of the implementation: the degree to which it met the participant's needs; the likelihood that they would recommend it to others; the degree to which it helped them deal with their problems, and whether or not they would like to repeat it. The higher the perceived quality of the implementation, the lower the level of satisfaction (**Figure 4.7**)

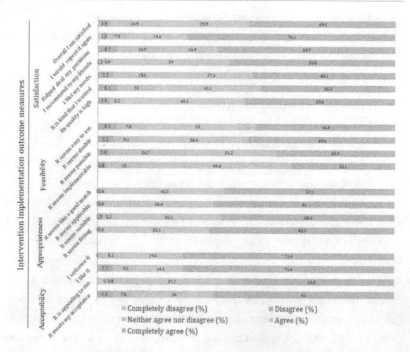

Figure 4. 7: Percentage of intervention group participants' rating on the intervention implementation outcome measures.

Ratings are given by participants, with a minimum score of 5 and a maximum score of 20, with the mean and standard deviation being analyzed by gender, age group, and school grade, along with testing the significance of any differences (**Table 4.13**). There was no significant difference in the scores for the implementation outcome measures based on the gender of the participants (p ≤ 0.05). There was a significant age difference in the ratings of acceptability of the implementation (p=0.003), appropriateness of the implementation (p=0.027), the feasibility of the implementation (p=0.012), and satisfaction with the implementation (p=0.013), with participants aged 18–19 years rating the implementation more highly. The level of satisfaction participants reported varied significantly (p=0.016) depending on their school grade, with participants in grades 11 and 12 reporting higher levels of satisfaction. There was no significant difference in the scores given based on a person's gender when it came to the implementation outcome measures ($p \leq 0.05$).

Table 4.13: Differences in perceived intervention implementation outcome measures by gender, age group, and school grade.

Intervention Outcome measures	The expected range of mean scores	Mean (SD) score					
		Gender		Age group		School grade	
		Male	Female	15-17	18-19	9-10	11-12
Acceptability	5-20	18.12 (2.58)	17.88(2.73)	17.03(3.13)	18.79(1.86)	17.64(3.02)	18.39(2.14)
		p= 0.701		p= 0.003		p= 0.211	
Appropriateness	5-20	18.33(2.03)	18.12(2.16)	17.65(2.31)	18.69(1.77)	17.95(2.25)	18.53(1.87)
		p= 0.666		p= 0.027		p= 0.225	
Feasibility	5-20	17.00(2.49)	16.56(2.62)	16.00(2.85)	17.44(2.09)	16.36(2.60)	17.26(2.42)
		p= 0.453		p= 0.012		p= 0.119	
Satisfaction	7-35	30.65(4.14)	289.53(4.94)	28.74(4.58)	31.28(4.18)	28.95(4.79)	31.40(3.91)
		p= 0.282		p= 0.013		p= 0.016	

4.3.4.2. Perceived Factors Influencing the Effectiveness and Implementation Outcomes

Lack of resources and one's personal and family-related challenges were the most likely factors to affect the perceived outcome measures of the implementation process (**Figure 4.8**). The primary focus of the analysis was the proportion of participants who responded "agree" or "completely agree" with each item. Most participants (71.5 %) reported that they did not have access to technological resources such as smartphones or computers; 77.9 % said they did not have easy internet access, and 72.7% reported poor internet coverage.

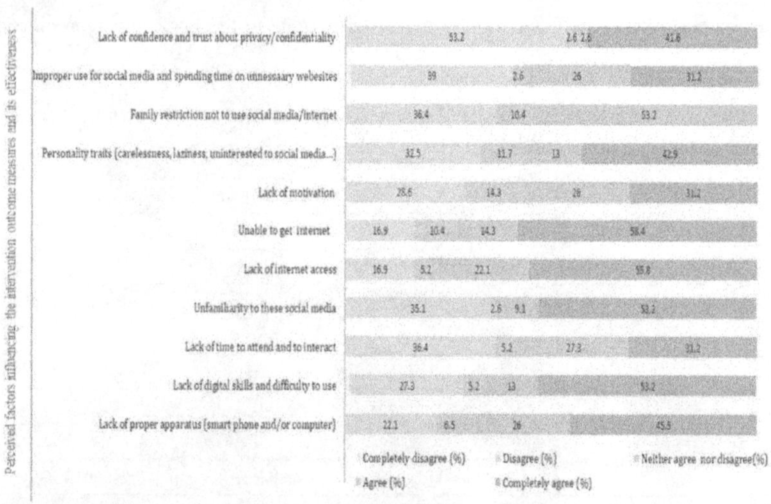

Figure 4. 8: Self-ratings of agreement with factors supposedly influencing the intervention implementation outcomes.

Personal factors such as a lack of time to engage with the intervention (58.5%), unfamiliarity with social media (62.3%), a lack of digital skills and difficulty using technology (66.2%), and a lack of motivation (57.2%), were less common but were still reported by over half of the respondents. Other reported factors included laziness or carelessness, or having little interest in social media (55.9%); misusing social media or spending time on unnecessary websites (57.2%); a lack of confidence and trust in the privacy or confidentiality of the intervention (44.2%); and a lack of confidence and trust in the privacy or confidentiality of the intervention. A restriction imposed by their families that prevented them from using social media or the internet (53.2%) was another factor that played a role.

Chapter Summary

The result section of the thesis is organized into the order of objectives. The presentation of findings for the part I of the thesis (cross-sectional) is followed by part II of the thesis (intervention). The cross-sectional(part-I) of the thesis includes (i) socio-demographic characteristics, (ii) mental health literacy level, (iii) the socio-demographics effect, (iv) self–reported mental health issues, the associated socio-demographic factors, and (v) the correlation of self–reported mental health issues and mental health literacy among school adolescents in an urban Ethiopia are reported. In the second part of the study (part-II), the effect size and difference-in-difference analysis have been demonstrated to investigate the intervention's effectiveness and success in improving adolescents' mental health literacy. Within this section of the thesis, the secondary analysis explored the four measures of the outcomes of the intervention's implementation: the implementation acceptability, the implementation appropriateness, the implementation feasibility, and the satisfaction of the intervention participant adolescents. Furthermore, the perceived factors affecting the intervention effectiveness and these measures' implementation outcome are reported.

The mean score of mental health literacy was normally distributed (Skewness=-1.321, Kurtosis=2.804) with a mean of 135.98 and SD=15.50; these scores were affected by socio-demographic characteristics. Males had slightly lower levels of mental health literacy (133.84) than females (138.12) (p<0.01). Regarding the formal normality test, skewness and kurtosis of the distribution are preferable over the eyeball test for both small and large samples. The formal normality tests (skewness and kurtosis) were preferred over the eyeball test to evaluate the normality of the data distribution. An asymmetric distribution is said to have skewness, while a peak distribution is said to have kurtosis. We use a skewness absolute value of less than two or a kurtosis absolute value of less than 7 for determining the substantial normality that the present findings fulfilled[278].

The mental health literacy score presented by graphs showed an absolute skew value far less than two and the absolute kurtosis (proper) far less than seven. When taken together, 10.7% variance in the mental health literacy of female adolescents and 8.9% of the variability in the mental health literacy of male adolescents accounted for the ethnicity/cultural affiliation, school grade, and level of parental education.

Prevalence of perceived mental health difficulties (total difficulties, internalizing, emotional problems and peer relationship problems) were higher viz. total difficulties 20%(15.9-25.5%), internalizing problems(14.9-28.4%), emotional problems(10.4-23.9%), and peer relationship problems(17.8-25.8%). It showed that these mental health difficulties were more serious for female adolescents than male adolescents. The most common mental health issue is depression, often measured by the well-being index (WHO-5) per the depression (ICD-10) inventory. A raw score of less than 13 or a score of 0 or 1 on any five items on the well-being index (WHO-5) is the cut-off score for depression (ICD-10). It was higher (25.5%) for female adolescents within 14-16 years.

A statistically significant association ($p \leq 0.05$) was observed between certain socio-demographic variables and these perceived mental health outcomes. When compared to the upper secondary grade level, the perceived mental health casenes prevalence was significantly higher for females in upper elementary (AOR: 2.60 (0.95-7.10) and lower secondary levels (AOR: 2.73(1.19-6.29)). However, there was no significant difference in the prevalence of mental health problems among males. It was significantly higher among adolescents who had either themselves or family members used psychoactive substances ($p \leq 0.05$). This increased risk was shown in both cases. However, there was no apparent age, parental educational level, or work position-related difference in the prevalence of mental health problems ($p > 0.05$). The research found a substantial negative correlation between mental health literacy levels and strength difficulties ratings. Conversely, mental health literacy levels were significantly associated with subjective mental well-being. Nonetheless, the strength of these correlation coefficients was weaker than expected. Both the intervention's effect size and the difference-in-differences estimates were positive numbers. Despite the age and gender disparities, the effect size was significantly more prominent in the intervention group than in the group that served as the control group ($p \leq 0.05$). The effect size was estimated by Cohen's d and Hedges' g values, which were medium to large ($d/g=0.429-0.767$, $p \leq 0.05$). Despite gender, age, and school grade differences, the difference-in-differences estimate reflected a significant effect (DID=0.348, CI: 0.154-0.542, $p < 0.001$) in improving mental health literacy statistically. Despite various socio-demographic characteristics contributing to the uncertainty, the intervention program was evaluated as appropriate, feasible, acceptable, and satisfactory. Multiple perceived individual attributes, resources, and family-related factors were reported to influence the effectiveness of intervention and implementation outcome measures.

CHAPTER FIVE

DISCUSSION

CHAPTER FIVE

5. DISCUSSION

This chapter focuses on the thesis's findings and discussion of previous related study results. Moreover, the strengths and limitations of the thesis were presented. The discussion was made on finding with previously published related findings on the theoretical, conceptual, empirical, and methodological evidence related to the study variables and contexts.

The mental health literacy of school adolescents in Dire Dawa, Ethiopia, was assessed along with the effect of socio-demographic characteristics. The mental health literacy score was normally distributed (Skewness=-1.321, Kurtosis=2.804) with a mean of 135.98 and SD=15.50. The mental health literacy level was reportedly affected by socio-demographic characteristics. An absolute skew value less than two or an absolute kurtosis (proper) less than seven is used as reference values for determining the substantial normality that the present findings fulfilled[278]. An asymmetric distribution is said to have skewness, while a peak distribution is said to have kurtosis. As far as the formal normality test is concerned, skewness(a measure of the asymmetry) and kurtosis(a measure of the peakedness) of the distribution are preferable over the eyeball test for both small and large samples[278]. The formal normality tests (skewness and kurtosis) were preferred over the eyeball test to evaluate the normality of the data distribution[278].

The findings supported the hypothesis that these socio-demographic characteristics strongly correlate with the level of mental health literacy possessed by adolescents and are in line with those reported elsewhere in the world[262,265,289–292]. These findings add to the handful of quantitative studies that come from LMICs, Ethiopia included.

Adolescents' backgrounds and socio-demographic characteristics are reportedly related to perceived mental health difficulty scales and levels of mental health literacy [71–73]. Age, gender, religious background, ethnicity, in some instances related to cultural perspectives, parental educational status, economic level, and access to information like social media are important factors. Self or parental use of the psychoactive substance also has a determinant role[71,73,293].

According to the results of this research, the pattern of the mental health literacy levels among male and female adolescents differed significantly. The findings of this study were consistent with those of other reported results in that female participants had slightly higher levels of mental health literacy (mean=138.12±13.59) than male participants (mean=133.64±16.95). For instance, one study found that female Portuguese adolescents had reportedly higher scores of mental health literacy(mean=132.68 ±10.64) than their male counterparts (mean = 130.49±11.80)[262]. This was determined by comparing the two groups' means. Among students in Australia[60], and the USA[265,289], gender differences in mental health literacy have been observed, with studies consistently reporting lower mental health literacy among male participants. According to another nationwide survey conducted in the United States, males have a more pessimistic outlook than females regarding help-seeking behaviours associated with mental illness [290].

Other socio-demographic factors and the gender gap in mental health literacy levels contributed to the difference. Further research showed that these factors affect male and female participants differently[294]. There was a correlation between a person's mental health literacy and their ethnicity or cultural affiliation, school grade, and the level of education their parents had. These factors together accounted for 10.7% of the variability in the mental health literacy of female adolescents and 8.9% in the mental health literacy of male adolescents.

The finding was consistent with a report that health-related knowledge and deprived health information among children and adolescents in Ethiopia indicated variation across age groups, gender, culture, and provinces[8]. Other related previous studies also reported similar evidence[24,295,296]. However, this suggests that these factors only account for a relatively minor contribution to the variation in mental health literacy. This highlights the necessity of gaining an understanding of the influence that is exerted by other factors.

Schooling has significantly impacted adolescents' mental health literacy[265,289]. A recent study in the United States, for example, revealed that adolescents in lower grades had lower levels of mental health literacy[297]. Middle-school Chinese adolescents had higher mental health literacy than primary-school students, and college students had even higher[298]. The current study supported these findings. The mental health literacy level was associated with school grade, which was especially significant in female adolescents (p<0.01). School grade accounted for approximately 2.4% and 1.0% of the variability in mental health literacy among female and male adolescents, respectively, with a similar pattern of gender variation as previously discussed.

Individuals' knowledge, attitudes, and beliefs about mental health issues have been influenced by their ethnicity and cultural affiliations[290,297,299,300]. Cultural factors are closely related to race and ethnicity, with disparities in attitudes toward mental illness and adherence to mental health services[300]. When addressing mental health literacy in countries with multicultural and multiethnic diversity, such as Ethiopia, it is essential to demonstrate an understanding of cultural differences.

It is nonetheless surprising that mental health issues, mental health literacy, and socio-demographic factors have barely been investigated. Gender, age, education level, ethnicity/culture/religion, and family history have little effect on adolescent mental health literacy[90]. However, despite the scarcity of empirical data and contexts, studies reveal that mental health literacy level differs by gender, age, education level, ethnicity/culture, religious affiliation, and parental education level[98].

The current study found an association between one's ethnicity or cultural affiliation and their level of mental health literacy. This association accounts for 6.5 %and 6.1% of the variability in mental health literacy in female and male adolescents, respectively. A person's ethnic/cultural affiliation is the single most crucial factor in determining willingness to use mental health services[297]. From the present study, connections to the Oromo (p<0.01), the Somali (p<0.01), or another ethnicity/culture ethnic affiliation (p< 0.01) were negatively associated with mental health literacy when compared to people with Amhara ethnic/cultural affiliation. The belief that norms and shared cultural values aligned with a person's racial or ethnic identity strongly influence social conventions, psychological processes, and behaviour may be related to these associations [300]. In the context of Ethiopia, ethnic and cultural affiliation is strongly intertwined with religious affiliation and vice versa. A person's religious affiliation tends to dictate their beliefs, attitudes, and behaviours in many other aspects of life, affecting their mental health literacy and mental health outcomes[301]. An individual's beliefs, exposures, knowledge, and behaviour regarding health determinants and outcomes are determined by the collections of practices, rituals, and beliefs they engage in that are underpinned by the same spiritual values [302]. Previous studies have found significant and positive associations between religious involvement and mental health, with higher levels of social support and a lower prevalence of substance abuse [303]. Spirituality and religious participation have been shown to impact mental health outcomes positively[305]. Praying and reading material with a spiritual focus can give people who have actively involved in religious practices the impression of being connected to a higher power, which can boost their mood positively[305].

In a similar vein, these people may have a more positive social influence as a result of their religious practice, which in turn raises awareness about issues of mental health [304]. This could make them more likely to live healthy lifestyles. Positive psychological and physical health outcomes have been reported from communities with high participation in faith-based organizations, where religious activities, in many cases, serve as an alternative source of support and treatment for individuals who struggle with mental ill-health [305]. It has been found that religious belief is related to positive emotions, and it has also been found that people who have firmly held religious beliefs experience more positive emotions than those who are less religious [304]. Research conducted on Protestants and Catholics found a significant link between higher levels of spirituality, social support, and overall life satisfaction[303]. Differences in religious doctrine and how religious doctrine is communicated are two of the many factors that influence how different religions approach psychology and mental health. For instance, a study of Protestants, Jews, and Catholics revealed a correlation between social support and the prominence of specific mental states in all three religious groups[304]. This finding was consistent across all three religious traditions. On the other hand, the connection between spirituality, religious belief, and coping mechanisms was stronger in Catholics and Protestants than in Jews[304].

There was a correlation that could be considered statistically significant between mental health literacy and the levels of education attained by parents. It is commonly demonstrated that parents are regulators of their children's well-being and play a significant role in facilitating their children's mental health literacy and mental health outcomes. As a result, the attitude of adolescents toward mental health treatment is strongly correlated with their parental education level[290], which is likely also reflected in the perspectives of their children. According to the findings of this study, adolescent males and females have different relationships regarding the level of mental health literacy associated with their parental education level. This relationship accounts for 2.1% and 2.0% of the variance in mental health literacy of female and male adolescents, respectively. There is evidence to suggest that similar associations exist. For instance, a study conducted in Sri Lanka found that adolescents whose mothers had completed some level of postsecondary education had the lowest mental health literacy score, which is in line with the findings of the present investigation[92]. These effects may be because educated mothers often have significant work commitments. As a result, they have less time to spend with their children during the crucial mental and emotional development stages, which can be one of the possible justifications for this phenomenon.

The correlation between mental health literacy level, the strength difficulty scale, and mental well-being scores was reported. It showed mental health literacy negatively correlated with strength difficulties scores and positively associated with mental well-being; both were significantly but weaker in magnitude. The findings of this study were in agreement with previous findings and theories. For instance, a study demonstrated that the depression prevalence was 1.52 times among individuals with inadequate mental health literacy, implying a clear negative association between mental health literacy and depression[98]. Another study depicted mental health literacy as an explanatory variable of the mental well-being of adolescents having a positive correlation with it[306].

Strength difficulties scores predict mental disorder prevalence across the adolescent population's backgrounds. Cross-cultural comparisons require great caution[307]. The baseline for cut-off scores definition of total and subscales difficulty scores were taken from the United Kingdom population norms defined during the instrument development [112,308]. These cut-off scores were validated in several studies from the global and African contexts[91,271,309–313]. The cut-off score for the present study was slightly lower for total difficulties and hyperactivity scores than the baseline and relatively higher for an internalizing score; these were almost the same as the baseline definition (**Table 4.5**). Some evidence indicated that lower cut-off values have been more effective than the higher cut-off values at identifying the perceived mental health difficulties of children and adolescents[313]. However, local cut-off values are required to ensure cultural, epidemiological, and demographic equivalence[272]. Hence, the cut-off score ranges from the present study implied the need for a newer cut-off range for both the original 3-band and 4-band categorizations. Similarly, an appraisal of the reliability test, validation, and use of SDQ in Africa revealed the importance of cultural, epidemiological and demographic equivalence of local cut-off scores in various assessment settings[272].

The present study's finding was within the same range of the Ethiopian national level prevalence of adolescent mental health problems, reportedly ranging from 17-23%[78], with other study results in the Ethiopian context[9,85,150]. Prevalence of total difficulties (15.9-25.5%), internalizing problem (14.9-28.4%), emotional problem (10.4-23.9%), and peer relationship problem (17.8-25.8%) was similar that was within the range of global prevalence(10-20%)[28].

Several studies showed that discrepancies were observed from one region to another and from one country to another[149,314–316]. Similarly, there is a difference in the prevalence of mental health issues among adolescent male and female adolescents[151]. In this study, the female gender was significantly associated with total difficulty score, consistent with a finding among Indian children[314]. Being female was comparatively linked with better mental health outcomes[314]. A study among children and adolescents from seven European countries (Netherlands, Italy, Turkey, Germany, Bulgaria, Romania, and Lithuania) reported that externalized problems were consistently higher in males than females and reversed for internalized problems[149]. Another study from South Africa showed that the proportion of females with emotional symptoms, total difficulties, and pro-social behavioural problems was higher than their male counterparts.

In contrast, conduct and hyperactivity-inattention problems were significantly more severe among males than females[281]. Consistent with other studies, the prevalence of conduct and externalizing problems was more significant among male adolescents than females. For example, a study in Northeast china showed a similar result[151].

One possible explanation for that might be that mental health issues are influenced by the cultural, economic, and geographical environments in which individuals live[315]. These conditions lead to inequalities that disproportionally affect gender differences and are heavily associated with risk factors for many common mental disorders[315]. According to the WHO, the relationship between the mental health problems prevalence and poverty indices was statistically significant[316]. These poverty indices are education disparity, low income, lack of material goods, lack of job, and housing obstacles. For several cultural and traditional reasons, these factors impact females more than boys [316].

Odds of mental health problems were significantly associated with some socio-demographic characteristics (p<0.05) differing in magnitude across these characteristics. The mental health problems prevalence was considerably higher for females in upper elementary and lower secondary levels than for upper secondary grade levels (p<0.05), consistent with reports of several studies. WHO reported educational levels as essential for adolescent mental health issues[316].

However, the difference was insignificant for male adolescents. Furthermore, differences in prevalence have existed but little across the three age groups, maternal and paternal education level, and job types or level of employment (p>0.05). From the current study, the proportion of adolescents with reported perceived mental health problems was two times higher among adolescents with a self and/or family members' experience of psychoactive substance use (p<0.05). On the contrary, a finding from Northeast China revealed that the prevalence of any mental disorders and internalizing disorders was significantly lower in younger adolescents than elders[151]. The highest proportion of children from the same population aged 11–14 had reported internalizing problems than any age group[151].

Mental health literacy positively correlates with mental well-being and negatively correlates with strength difficulties scores. These findings were consistent with existing theories and results of previous studies[91,317–319]. However, the magnitudes of the correlation coefficient were lower. The scarcity of skilled professionals and facilities increases the mental health promotion and prevention gap in developing countries[91,317–319]. Hence, there exist barriers and difficulties in accessing treatment for mental health problems from economic(cost and financial limitation) and health providers' side(prejudice, ill-treatment, and bias)[320]. Another possible explanation is that the well-established effect of low health literacy on poor physical and mental health issues might determine the proposed relationship through the mediation effect of self-efficacy[321].

Mental health literacy significantly influences adolescents' perceptions and emotional responses[322], reflecting perceived mental health issues and subjective mental well-being. Several studies revealed that mental health literacy had a significant relationship with mental health issues[194,323,324]. A higher level of mental well-being has been reported among adolescents with better know-how about obtaining mental health services[322]. Adolescents' awareness of symptoms, causes, and mental illness treatment contributes to favourable and positive attitudes toward seeking help[48]. Similarly, adolescents with better mental health literacy are less likely to engage in problematic health behaviours[122]. They have better self-efficacy and help-seeking intention, leading to better mental health and well-being[122].

Of course, help-seeking intention and self-efficacy may reflect only one of several mechanisms. Better mental health literacy leads to better mental well-being. Higher help-seeking intention and self-efficacy would only partially mediate the relation between higher mental health literacy and better mental well-being. Components of health behaviour expressed in actions, targets, contexts, and time are the most determining factors of mental health outcomes[325,326].

Mental health literacy influences the perceived and expected mental health services for the perceived and anticipated need for treatment[88], indicating the need to integrate mental health literacy and help-seeking. Hence, mental health literacy is essential to improve and often but not always corresponds to help-seeking behaviours[187]. Anthony F. Jorm and his colleagues revealed that changing knowledge in principle is vital and not problematic; however, changing heartily emotional reactions to practice caring and preventing mental disorders may be much harder[23].

Help-seeking, interchangeably health-seeking, has become one of the essential perspectives in understanding causes and factors for patient delay from appropriate action across different health conditions[94]. Despite the prevalent mental health problems and poor well-being, adolescents' unwillingness and low intention to seek help usually result in delays in timely treatment[90]. Most adolescents with mental health problems are reluctant and miss the use of healthcare for mental health, which increases the complexity of social, mental, and general health outcomes[327]. The findings presented from this study implied that promoting mental health literacy can improve subjective mental well-being[322].

Effect size and difference-in-difference analysis were used throughout the intervention portion of the study to examine a mental health curriculum intervention effectiveness that was delivered using social media to enhance adolescent mental health literacy. The secondary analysis looked at the intervention implementation acceptability, feasibility, appropriateness, and the beneficiaries' level of satisfaction with the program. Additionally, the perceived factors that affect the intervention effectiveness and measure these implementation outcomes were evaluated.

Mental health literacy is a modifiable factor explained in terms of individuals' knowledge, beliefs, and awareness about mental health issues[17,20–23]. These factors increase self-efficacy, the likelihood of seeking help, and encourage healthy behaviours, which ultimately contribute to mental well-being and good mental health[29,49]. The effects of these changes can be either immediate or intermediate, and their consequences can be characterized as either proximal or distal[59].

The study's findings revealed that the intervention effect was far more remarkably greater than zero, and the magnitude of the impact was demonstrated using the standardized metrics of effect size and difference-in-differences estimate. Compared to a control condition, the intervention had a significantly more significant impact ($p<0.05$), as measured by both the effect size and the difference-in-differences analysis. However, the magnitudes of these measures depend considerably on the participant's gender and age. Despite several factors that affected the implementation of the intervention that varied depending on the participants' socio-demographic characteristics, the intervention was acceptable, appropriate, feasible, and satisfactory.

Conventional and comparison approaches are two ways to interpret effect size outcomes for quantitative intervention analyses[114,115,286,328]. However, the vast majority of currently available evidence recommends using the conventional approach for studies such as this one with little previously available evidence for comparison[285]. The effect size is typically presented in Cohen's d and/or Hedges' g values when using the conventional statistical analysis method that divides it into three ranges of magnitude: small (below 0.2), medium (0.2 to 0.5), and large (0.5 or higher)[285]. The estimate of the intervention's effect size in this study was significant and more remarkably greater than zero; the intervention program may have improved the adolescents' mental health literacy. The effect size observed in this study would be conventionally classified as moderate to high, with a difference across gender and age groups. The effect size of the present study(d=0.429-0.767, p<0.05) was consistent with the findings of a previously published meta-analysis on universal and selective intervention studies to improve mental health literacy that included a mental health curriculum intervention(d=0.541-0.774, p<0.05)[50]. This finding was consistent with a report from a meta-analysis of digital interventions improving positive mental health outcomes among young people involving supervision (Cohen's d=0.52) and without involvement supervision (Cohen's d = 0.33) [329] despite little evidence in the Ethiopian context for further comparison.

The coefficient of the estimated difference-in-differences reflects that this intervention study has had a higher and more significant impact, according to the results obtained from regression models stratified by gender and age group (p<0.001). Despite some differences, the intervention significantly increased overall mental health literacy across all age groups and genders. Therefore, the mental health curriculum intervention that was carried out using social media greatly improved adolescents' mental health literacy, supporting the initial hypothesis. Previous qualitative research has demonstrated that online health interventions have successfully overcome various obstacles and challenges related to logistics and the physical environment[86].

Although there was little quantitative evidence available for comparison, the results of this study were consistent with those of earlier qualitative studies[86]. It has been demonstrated that socio-demographic and socio-economic factors can affect the effectiveness and outcomes of health interventions[330]. For instance, numerous studies have shown that gender dynamics affect the outcomes of efforts to change the health-related behaviours of children and adolescents[331]. As a result, the regression models for the present study's analysis were stratified after multiple observable confounders. These confounders were controlled for by determining the significance of the variability in mental health literacy across these different groups. For instance, a previous study on Ethiopia's population found that girls had slightly better awareness of mental health issues than boys[106]. It was consistent with other related studies carried out in Australia,

Portugal, and the United States of America[262,265,289]. In addition, the effectiveness of this study's mental health literacy intervention differed by sex and age, regardless of the methods used to measure that effectiveness. The difference-in-difference estimate was higher among girls than boys, and the effect size was higher for participants aged 15-17 years ($p<0.05$).

Age is a factor that can be associated with the results of health interventions[332]. According to results from this investigation, the effect of the intervention on the mental health literacy scores as estimated with difference-in-differences (DID) was significantly greater for older adolescents than younger adolescents. One plausible explanation is that older adolescents devote more time and attention to the activities they participate in than younger adolescents do. Younger adolescents may have a shorter ability to focus and pay attention for a more extended length of time[54]. Differences in adolescents' cognitive and behavioural skills have also been shown to affect the outcomes of such interventions [54].

There was a significant difference in the participant ratings of the perceived outcome measures of the intervention implementation process across age groups ($p<0.05$), with older adolescents reporting closer to complete agreement with the implementation outcome measures. This effect of age may be explained by the difference in using technology, accessing the internet, and having digital literacy. It's possible that older adolescents will have more accessible opportunities and time accessing the internet and will have a higher level of digital literacy. These findings were consistent with those of previous similar studies[240,333].

The present findings found that the participants' demographic characteristics significantly contributed to the variation of the level of perceived intervention implementation outcome measures. Related study reports have shown that participant sex is one of the essential factors in predicting internet use behaviour[333]. In this regard, females are more receptive to digital interventions for behaviour change than males; because they reportedly spend more time on social media[333]. Nevertheless, there was no significant gender difference in the ratings of implementation outcome measures in the present study in contrast to earlier reports[240,333,334]. These findings, therefore, require further quantitative evidence from the wider population and in-depth qualitative explanations.

This study further investigated several perceived factors that were claimed to impact the effectiveness of intervention and implementation outcome measures. These perceived factors that influence the intervention effectiveness and measures of implementation outcome, among others, include (1) personal factors (confidence, digital skills, privacy concerns, interaction frequency to the internet or social media, motivation, use of other unnecessary websites, and personality traits), (2) lack of access to resources (access to devices and the internet), (3) family-related factors (being prohibited from accessing social media or the internet). Lack of apparatus (45.5%), poor digital skill (53.2%), and lack of internet access (58.8%) were relatively the most perceived factors influencing the implementation outcomes (Figure 4.8). Findings from the current study were consistent with the reports of other related studies of digital or web-based interventions[335–339]; in which adherence[338], participant engagement[339], and lack of money or internet access[337], were revealed to be associated with the effectiveness of an intervention. Behavioral factors[335] and digital or internet literacy[336] were also reported to be related to the effectiveness of an intervention. Understanding the participant's concerns and motivation is essential in developing successful web-based or digitally-based intervention programs[340].

Strengths and Limitations of the Study

Like any other scientific study, the present research likely has its strengths and limitations. The potential strength of the thesis was that it was a new study in Ethiopia, to the best of the scholar's knowledge, to introduce such mental health literacy investigation and intervention study using social media as a communication channel. The publications of findings from the study are an example and a reference to the mental health literacy body of knowledge in developing countries. A robust study protocol and procedures were followed. The sample size determination, sampling, and data collection procedures followed strict protocol with explicit inclusion and inclusion criteria. The data collection tools were pre-existing tools validated for the same population age group and validated this study context. The data were collected by trained individuals with basic know-how about basic concepts of health sciences and experience related to data collection with utmost supervision. The study was conducted in a real-life natural environment with a relatively lower cost of implementation, reducing potential confounders with the possible advantage of improved external validity[341]. The reliability of the statistical analysis was high.

This study's outcomes significantly contribute to the existing literature about interventions to improve adolescents' mental health literacy and intervention implementation outcome measures. First, the availability of such quantitative evidence in the form of standardized effect sizes and difference-in-difference estimates presents an opportunity to demonstrate further practical significance than the statistical significance and impact of digital and web-based interventions promoting adolescent mental health literacy. Second, it provides quantitative data for researchers interested in drawing meta-analytic conclusions and comparing with other related studies expressed using effect sizes and difference-in-difference analyses. Third, these findings reported in terms of the effect size and difference-in-difference contribute to the design and planning of new studies, including estimating required sample sizes with the desired likelihood.

The study has some inherent limitations. One of the study's potential limitations was the difficulty of generalizing study results to all adolescents (10-19 years) because the samples were selected from the age group(11-19) and grade level (5-12) that adolescents at the age of 10 years were in the first cycle elementary schools excluded during schools sampling. Likewise, the adolescents who participated in the intervention study were aged 15-19 years, with reasonable criteria that impact the generalizability of findings. Like any other study involving a quasi-experimental design, these findings could be influenced by various types of bias. One of the potential thesis limitations was the lack of previously available reliable empirical evidence involving interventions of this kind, restricted quantitative comparison efforts, and a highly restricted approach to the conventional interpretation of the effect size. The choices made in adopting the present study perspectives and the interpretations process may produce bias in study findings given the vivid debate on global/public mental health as well as health literacy perspectives and their interpretations.

During the conversation, although ethical approval and consent were guaranteed, information privacy might be considered a possible limitation that challenges the ethical consideration. Social media contamination was another anticipated limitation, even though the due emphasis was given throughout the study. The overwhelming cultural difference and other moderators were not considered.

Chapter Summary

The present study's findings contribute to the lack of quantitative evidence gap in low-income countries, particularly Ethiopia, due to its potential limitations. The mental health literacy score was normally distributed with variation across socio-demographic-related factors. The findings ascertained that adolescent mental health literacy significantly correlated with socio-demographic background, consistent with earlier findings worldwide. The relationship was statistically significant between adolescents' ethnicity or cultural affiliation and their level of mental health literacy. Ethnicity/cultural affiliation accounted for approximately 6.5% and 6.1% of the variation in the level of mental health literacy of male and female adolescents, respectively. Generalizing these findings should be by caution due to cultural differences. Despite insufficient studies on mental health literacy, the proportion of adolescents suffering from mental illness and poor mental health has increased. Adolescents suffer disproportionately from mental health issues compared to other age groups.

The intervention effectiveness reported in effect size and difference in difference estimate was significantly greater than zero; that suggests that the intervention program has the potential to improve adolescents' mental health literacy. Despite some differences, the intervention significantly increased mental health literacy scores across all ages and genders. Hence, the intervention of mental health curriculum implemented using social media significantly improved adolescents' mental health literacy, supporting the original hypothesis. The study revealed that the perceived outcome measures of the intervention process rated by study participants were somewhat different across age groups ($p<0.05$). Older adolescent groups agreed more strongly with the implementation outcome measures than the younger adolescents.

This study further investigated several perceived factors that were claimed to affect the effectiveness of intervention and implementation outcome measures. These perceived factors, among others, include (1) personal factors (confidence, digital skills, privacy concerns, interaction frequency to the internet or social media, motivation, use of other unnecessary websites, and personality traits), (2) lack of access to resources (access to devices and the internet), (3) family-related factors (being prohibited from accessing social media or the internet). Findings from the current study were consistent with the reports of other related studies of digital or web-based interventions.

CHAPTER SIX

CONCLUSION, IMPLICATION, AND FUTURE PROSPECTS

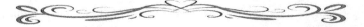

CHAPTER SIX
CONCLUSION, IMPLICATIONS, AND FUTURE PROSPECTS

This chapter focuses on the thesis's conclusion, implications, and prospects for future research. These subheadings under this chapter are the following.

- Conclusion
- Implications of the Thesis
- Prospects for Future Research

6.1. Conclusion

This study is probably the first-hand study in Ethiopia that mainly looked into the mental health literacy of junior and high school adolescents. The scope and the overarching aims of this thesis primarily were to examine (1) mental health literacy level,(2) the perceived mental health issues, and (3) the effective intervention of mental health curriculum using social media to improve the mental health literacy of adolescents in Dire Dawa city, Ethiopia. It comprised two consecutive phases of study designs: cross-sectional and quasi-experimental designs. These findings highlighted empirical evidence that had not previously been prominent in the literature from Africa and Ethiopia[342,343]. It would contribute to filling the evidence gap in the availability of quantitative evidence about the mental health literacy level of adolescents from low-income countries, most notably in the African context, particularly Ethiopia. While recognizing some limitations of the study, the present thesis has primarily achieved the proposed research questions, hypotheses, and objectives through the lens of the revised theory of integrated health behavior change model and theory of change the findings presented in chapter four.

The first expected outcome of the thesis (*Objective 1*) from the study's first phase examined adolescents' mental health literacy level and the effect of some socioeconomic factors. The mental health literacy score was normally distributed (Skewness=-1.321, Kurtosis=2.804) with a mean score of 135.98 and a standard deviation of 15.50[106]. These scores were affected by socio-demographic characteristics. The socio-demographic factors have affected the mental health literacy of adolescents. For instance, mental health literacy score was slightly higher among female adolescents than male adolescents. When taken together, adolescents' ethnic/cultural affiliation, school grade, and the educational level of their parents accounted for approximately one-tenth (~10%) of the variation in their mental health literacy. These effects were nearly similar for both female and male adolescents.

The second expected outcome of the thesis (*Objective 2*) from the study's first phase revealed adolescents' perceived mental health issues and the effect of some socio-demographic factors. It was achieved using the same sample of adolescents using the commonly employed tools, namely the strength difficulty questionnaire (SDQ) and mental well-being index (WHO-5). The strength difficulty cut-off score for the present study was slightly lower for total strength difficulty and hyperactivity scores than the baseline despite relatively higher internalizing scores implying these cut-off scores were almost the same as the baseline definition. The finding was within the same range as the Ethiopian national level prevalence of adolescent mental health problems, reportedly ranging from 17-23%. The prevalence of rate of total difficulties (15.9-25.5%), internalizing problems (14.9-28.4%), emotional problems(10.4-23.9%), and peer relationship problems (17.8-25.8%) were similar that was slightly within the range of the global prevalence(10-20%). As depicted from strength difficulties scores, the perceived mental health problems were significantly associated with some socio-demographic characteristics (p<0.05) differing in magnitude.

Female adolescents scored higher on the total difficulties and subscale difficulties than their male counterparts. Perceived mental health issues prevalence was significantly higher for females in upper elementary and lower secondary levels than for upper secondary grade levels (p<0.05), consistent with reports of several studies. Furthermore, differences in prevalence have existed but little across the three age groups, maternal and paternal education level, and job types or level of employment (p>0.05). An analysis of the present study's mental health prevalence was twice higher among adolescents with a self and/or family members' experience of psychoactive substance use (p<0.05).

The third expected outcome of the thesis (*Objective 3*) from the study's first phase showed the correlation between mental health literacy level and the strength difficulty scale and mental well-being scores. It showed mental health literacy negatively correlated with strength difficulties scores and positively associated with mental well-being; both were significantly but weaker in magnitude. These findings were consistent with existing theories and results of previous studies.

The second phase of the thesis (a quasi-experimental study) aimed to test a proposed hypothesis of whether a mental health curriculum intervention using social media effectively improves adolescents' mental health literacy(*Objective 4*). Furthermore, it aimed to examine the status of implementation outcome measures (*Objective 5*) and perceived factors influencing these expected intervention outcomes (*Objective 6*).

The thesis supports the assertion that an intervention using an evidence-based mental health curriculum delivered via social media significantly improves the mental health literacy of adolescents[343]. Both the intervention's effect size and the difference-in-differences estimates were positive numbers. The effect size was estimated by Cohen's d and Hedges' g values, which were medium to large (d/g=0.429-0.767, p≤0.05). It was significantly more prominent in the group that received the intervention than the group that served as the control (p≤0.05)[343]. The difference-in-differences (DID) estimate reflected a significant effect (DID=0.348, CI:0.154-0.542,p<0.001) in improving mental health literacy with statistical significance[343]. The effect size and difference-in-differences estimate reflected that the intervention effectiveness differed with gender, age, and school grade[343].

We found that the implementation of the intervention was considered acceptable, appropriate, feasible, and satisfactory; despite the effects of various socio-demographic characteristics contributing to the uncertainty[343]. Multiple perceived individual attributes, resources, and family-related factors were reported to influence the effectiveness of intervention and implementation outcome measures. Generalizing these findings should be by caution due to cultural differences.

6.2. Implications of the Thesis

These findings' notation and significant implications are the inferences for public health practices promoting adolescents' mental health. The scientific reports from such studies contribute empirical evidence in contemplating the role of mental health literacy as a domain of good mental health and its interactions with some mental health outcomes and associated factors through the integrated theory of mental health behaviour change model. It has sought to make a significant contribution to understanding the mental health literacy level, (2) the perceived mental health issues, and (3) the effectiveness of mental health curriculum intervention using social media to improve the adolescents' mental health literacy level in Dire Dawa city, Ethiopia.

Socio-demographic factors contributed to the variation of mental health literacy levels and a significant proportion difference in adolescents' perceived mental health issues implying the necessity of considering these differences. It underscored the importance of understanding these socio-demographic factors contributing to the wide range of adolescents' mental health literacy and perceived mental health issues. Although these socio-demographic characteristics generally make a small contribution, gender-based and culturally congruent approaches are essential to enhance adolescents' mental health outcomes. These differences must be taken into account when designing interventions.

The strong positive correlations between mental health literacy and mental well-being and the considerably negative associations between strength difficulties scores and mental health literacy were consistent with existing theories and the findings of previous studies. It suggested the effects of mental health literacy on proximal and distal mental health outcomes through the lens of a contextualized integrated theory of mental health behaviour change model.

Adolescents' understanding of mental health issues was improved significantly due to the mental health curriculum intervention program delivered using guided social media platforms. Digital and online interventions for positive mental health promotion are feasible and scalable. Nevertheless, it is necessary to consider socio-demographic disparities and barriers to inclusion and compliance. When attempting to promote adolescents' mental health effectively, it is essential to consider the various levels of mental health literacy. Perceived influencing factors found to limit the success of the intervention implied the need to consider these determinates for effective adolescent mental health promotion using social media.

Promoting positive mental health through adolescents' mental health literacy domains should reflect and prioritize groups that start to have perceived mental health difficulties. Hence, it is recommended that the coordinated public health and education sector stakeholders contemplate mental health literacy in the schooling system and school mental health promotion packages. Use of internet facilities and platforms-most importantly, social media as mental health curriculum intervention platform for adolescent positive mental health promotion is recommended. It indicated the potential of scaling up such an intervention to exploit emerging digital and online outlets in promoting good mental health in general and mental health literacy of adolescents in particular.

6.3. Prospects for Future Research

A culturally congruent program is necessary for promoting adolescents' mental health through the constructs and contents of [mental] health literacy. Hence, it is essential to demonstrate an understanding of these differences in countries with multicultural and multiethnic diversity, such as Ethiopia. Therefore, further studies should envisage understanding the remaining factors explaining the mental health literacy of adolescents and its proximal and distal outcomes that affect the effectiveness and positive intervention outcomes. Future interventions should also consider other factors contributing to good mental health. Qualitative studies should involve unfolding how and why these happen.

Further studies need to be conducted on the mental health literacy of rural adolescents. The contextually integrated mental health behaviour change model includes autonomous motivation, attitude, biological, economic, and environmental factors. Hence, future research prospects need to consider these intrapersonal and interpersonal determinants of mental health literacy, such as self-efficacy, help-seeking intention, health behaviour, and interaction with mental health literacy.

Concerted and ongoing planning and engagement of adolescents for mental health promotion must consider multiple perspectives and approaches. Future interventions should consider other factors contributing to good mental health, including remaining socio-demographic and contextual factors.

Chapter Summary

The present study has largely achieved all the proposed research questions, hypotheses, and objectives through the lens of the revised theory of integrated health behavior change model and theory of change. The scores on mental health literacy were normally distributed, but the distribution changed depending on the socio-demographic factors.

A significant proportion of adolescents experienced mental health problems (15.9-28.4%) and were significantly associated with some socio-demographic characteristics(p<0.05) differing in magnitude (*Objective 2*). Mental health literacy negatively correlated with strength difficulties scores and positively related to mental well-being; both were significantly but weaker in magnitude (*Objective 3*). These findings were consistent with existing theories and results of previous studies.

Both the intervention's effect size and the difference-in-differences estimates were positive numbers. The implementation of the intervention was considered acceptable, appropriate, feasible, and satisfactory; despite the effects of various socio-demographic characteristics contributing to the uncertainty. Multiple perceived individual attributes, resources, and family-related factors were reported to influence the effectiveness of intervention and implementation outcome measures

The present study's findings underscore the importance of understanding the various factors contributing to the wide range of mental health literacy among adolescents. Gender-based and culturally congruent approaches are essential to enhance the mental health outcomes of adolescents.

It contributes empirical evidence in contemplating the role of mental health literacy as a domain of good mental health and its interactions with mental health outcomes and associated factors through the integrated theory of mental health behaviour change model.

Hence, it is recommended that the coordinated public health and education sector stakeholders contemplate mental health literacy in the schooling system and school mental health promotion packages. It indicated the potential of scaling up such an intervention to exploit emerging digital and online platforms in promoting good mental health in general and

It is essential to have a culturally congruent and relevant mental health literacy improvement initiative for successful mental health promotion. Hence, it is crucial to demonstrate an understanding of these differences in countries with multicultural and multiethnic diversity, such as Ethiopia, including rural adolescents. Therefore, further studies should envisage understanding the remaining factors explaining the mental health literacy of adolescents and its proximal and distal outcomes that affect the effectiveness and positive intervention outcomes. Future interventions should also consider other factors contributing to good mental health.

The contextually integrated mental health behaviour change model includes autonomous motivation, attitude, biological, economic, and environmental factors. Hence, the prospects of the present study need to consider these intrapersonal and interpersonal determinants of mental health literacy, such as self-efficacy, help-seeking intention, health behaviour, and interaction with mental health literacy. Thus, future interventions should consider other factors contributing to good mental health and socio-demographic and contextual factors. Hence, further qualitative studies should involve unfolding how and why these happen including other remaining determinants.